ApoB in Clinical Care

Cover and layout design: www.designworksnl.eu

ISBN 978 90 368 0979 5

J. de Graaf

P. Couture

A.D. Sniderman

ApoB

IN CLINICAL CARE

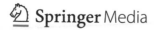 **Springer** Media   HOUTEN 2015

Table of contents

Foreword

This book was written for doctors who want to move forward, who want to give better care to their patients, and who are willing to learn how to do that. Accurate diagnosis is a core principle of clinical medicine but if only the conventional plasma and lipoprotein lipids are measured, accurate diagnosis of the atherogenic disorders of lipoprotein metabolism is not possible. Everything is reduced to one of three diagnoses: hypercholesterolemia, hypertriglyceridemia or mixed hypercholesterolemia and hypertriglyceridemia.

However, with measurement of total cholesterol, triglyceride and apoB and application of the apoB algorithm, with the exception of Lp(a), which requires a specific assay, accurate diagnosis of the apoB dyslipoproteinemias is now simple and fast.

Accurate diagnosis is the indispensable key to effective therapy for the individual patient and, as we demonstrate in this book, this principle certainly holds for the dyslipoproteinemias. Adding apoB to total cholesterol and triglyceride moves us from lipids to lipoprotein particles, from dyslipidemias to dyslipoproteinemias, from guessing what may be wrong to knowing what is wrong, from guessing what treatment should be best, to knowing which treatment is best, from just mindlessly following rules that others make, to understanding what to do and why you should do it.

With the apoB app, which is available for free in both the Apple App Store and Google Play Store, diagnosis takes only seconds and core material is immediately available. In this book, we integrate the relevant physiology, epidemiology and clinical trial results so that you can have a real understanding of how this new diagnostic and therapeutic approach works.

Cardiovascular disease is the commonest cause of death worldwide. Effective therapies are available but they need to be given to those who need them when the problem is recognized not after the complication has occurred.

This task has not been easy. Nothing worthwhile is. But without all the assistance we have received, we would not have come this far. Accordingly, we wish to thank all our colleagues who have encouraged us as well as our critics who have stimulated us. But, most of all, we want to record our infinite thanks and love for those who have believed in us and what we are trying to do, those who have supported us and loved us in all our moments of darkness, moments that seemed to stretch into eternity. They are the light that has kept us going.

This effort is imperfect. We acknowledge that. But we believe it is a step forward and forward is where we need to go if we are to improve the outcomes of our patients.

Jacqueline de Graaf
Patrick Couture
Allan Sniderman

About the authors

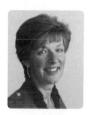

Prof. Dr. Jacqueline de Graaf, internist, FRCP
Department of Internal Medicine
Radboud university medical center,
Nijmegen, The Netherlands
jacqueline.degraaf@radboudumc.nl

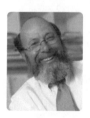

Prof. Dr. Allan Sniderman, cardiologist
Mike Rosenbloom Laboratory for Cardiovascular Research
McGill University Health Centre,
Montreal, Canada
allansniderman@hotmail.com

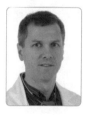

Prof. Dr. Patrick Couture, internist
Lipid Research Centre,
Laval University Medical Center,
Quebec City, Canada
patrick.couture@crchul.ulaval.ca

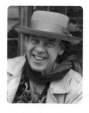

All the illustrations in this book were created by David Rolling.
The authors are so grateful to him.
david_rolling@sympatico.ca

List of abbreviations

ACAT	Acyl-CoA Cholesterol Acyltransferase
ALP	Atherogenic Lipoprotein Phenotype
apo	apolipoprotein
ASP	Acylation Stimulating Protein
ATPII	Adult Treatment Panel II
ARH	Autosomal Recessive Hypercholesterolemia
CAD	Coronary Artery Disease
CAPD	Continuous Ambulatory Peritoneal Dialysis
CETP	Cholesterol Ester Transfer Protein
CHD	Coronary Heart Disease
CR	Chylomicron Remnants
CTT	Cholesterol Treatment Trialists
CVD	Cardiovascular Disease
DM2	Type 2 Diabetes Mellitus
ERFC	Emerging Risk Factors Collaboration
ESRD	End-Stage Renal Disease
FA	Fatty Acids
FDB	Familial Defective ApoB100
FH	Familial Hypercholesterolemia
FCH	Familial Combined Hyperlipidemia
FDBL	Familial Dysbetalipoproteinemia
FHTG	Familial Hypertriglyceridemia
GPI	Glycophosphatidylinositol
HAART	Highly Active Antiretroviral Therapy
HDL-C	High Density Lipoprotein Cholesterol
HeFH	Heterozygous Familial Hypercholesterolemia
HIV	Human Immunodeficiency Virus
HoFH	Homozygous Familial Hypercholesterolemia
HPS	Heart Protection Study

HR	Hazard Ratio
HSP	Hormone Sensitive Lipase
IDL	Intermediate Density Lipoprotein
JBS	Joint British Societies
LCAT	Lecithin-Cholesterol Acyltransferase
LDL-C	Low Density Lipoprotein Cholesterol
LDL-P	Low Density Lipoprotein particle number
Lp(a)	Lipoprotein(a)
LPL	Lipoprotein Lipase
LRP	LDL-Receptor Related Protein
MTP	Microsomal Triglyceride Transfer Protein
NHANES	National Health and Nutrition Examination Survey
PCOS	Polycystic Ovary Syndrome
PCSK9	Proprotein Convertase Subtilisin Kexin Type 9
PUFA	Polyunsaturated Fatty Acids
RCT	Randomized Clinical Trial
RER	Rough endoplasmic reticulum
SER	Smooth endoplasmic reticulum
SLE	Systemic Lupus Erythematosus
SREBP	Sterol Regulatory Element Binding Protein
TC	Total Cholesterol
TG	Triglycerides
TSH	Thyroid-Stimulating Hormone
USF1	Upstream Stimulatory Factor 1
VLDL	Very Low Density Lipoprotein

Conversion of mmol/l to mg/dl

Cholesterol and triglyceride concentrations in mmol/l are converted to mg/dl by multiplying by 38.5 and 88.5, respectively.

1. The Life History of ApoB Lipoprotein Particles

1.1 Physiology of the ApoB Lipoprotein Particles

There are two families of apoB lipoprotein particles: the apoB48 lipoprotein particles and the apoB100 lipoprotein particles.

> **ApoB48 lipoprotein particles**
>
> The family of the apoB48 lipoprotein particles consists of chylomicrons and chylomicron remnants. Chylomicron particles are secreted by the intestine and each contains one molecule of apoB48. Initially, chylomicron particles transport dietary triglyceride to adipose tissue and muscle. Chylomicron remnants are the normal particles produced by removal of triglyceride by peripheral tissues from intact chylomicron particles and these normal remnant particles rapidly transport the residual triglyceride and all the dietary cholesterol to the liver.
>
> Chylomicron particles are too large to penetrate the arterial wall and very few are ever present in plasma at any given time. Accordingly, they do not increase the risk of vascular disease. However, if present in large excess, they do increase the risk of pancreatitis.
>
> By contrast, when their removal is markedly delayed in remnant lipoprotein disorder, the abnormal cholesterol-enriched chylomicron remnant particles that accumulate in large numbers increase atherogenic risk dramatically.

> **ApoB100 lipoprotein particles**
>
> The family of the apoB100 lipoprotein particles consists of VLDL, IDL, LDL and Lp(a) particles. VLDL and Lp(a) particles are secreted by the liver and each contains one molecule of apoB100. VLDL particles are converted into IDL particles, which are converted into LDL particles. With only a few exceptions, there are 9 times more LDL particles than VLDL particles and they are much smaller than VLDL particles and so they can penetrate the arterial wall much more easily. That is why LDL particles are so much more important in atherogenesis than VLDL particles. Similarly, there are almost always far more VLDL particles (10-fold more) than normal chylomicron or normal chylomicron remnant particles. LDL particles, IDL particles, Lp(a) particles and abnormal VLDL remnant particles are undoubtedly atherogenic whereas whether normal VLDL particles are highly atherogenic remains controversial.

1.1.1 Introduction

There are two families of apoB lipoprotein particles: the apoB48 lipoprotein particles and the apoB100 lipoprotein particles.[1-5] ApoB48 and apoB100 are proteins, which encircle the surface of a lipoprotein particle and provide the structural framework around which it is constructed. ApoB48 is a truncated version of apoB100[6] and, in humans, one molecule of apoB48 is present on every lipoprotein particle synthesized by the intestine whereas one molecule of the full-length protein, apoB100, is present on every lipoprotein particle synthesized and secreted by the liver. The principal members of the two families of apoB lipoprotein particles are illustrated in Figure 1.1.

The apoB48 lipoprotein particle family consists of chylomicrons and chylomicron remnants (CR). Chylomicrons are secreted by intestinal cells following a meal and transport the dietary lipids to target tissues within the body. Chylomicron particles are too large to penetrate the arterial wall with any facility and so accumulation of chylomicrons does not increase the risk of vascular disease. However, large numbers of intact chylomicron particles do increase the risk of pancreatitis. CR are chylomicron particles from which most of the triglyceride has been removed by adipose tissue and muscle but which still contain almost all the cholesterol. CR are normal particles present in small numbers in plasma, even in the postprandial period, because they are so rapidly removed by the liver.

   In remnant lipoprotein disorder, the removal of the normal CR particles is markedly delayed. Accordingly, large numbers of CR particles accumulate in plasma – 10 to 20 fold more than normal – and with their prolonged half-life in plasma, these become enriched in cholesterol. Unquestionably, atherogenic risk is markedly increased in this disorder and rapid, accurate diagnosis is one of the major practical advantages

FIGURE 1.1

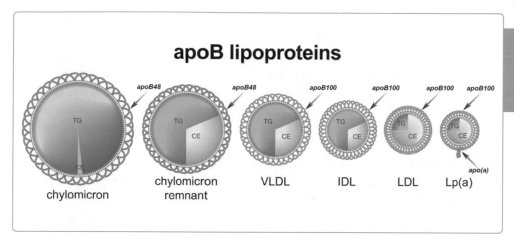

apoB lipoproteins

of the apoB algorithm. Whether atherogenic risk is significantly increased when CR removal is only slightly delayed and the number of remnant particles is only slightly increased remains controversial. In these situations, there are, on average, 10 times more very low-density lipoprotein (VLDL) particles than CR particles and generally 9 times more low-density (LDL) particles than VLDL particles.

The family of the apoB100 lipoprotein particles consists of VLDL, intermediate-density lipoprotein (IDL), LDL and Lp(a) particles. Each contains one molecule of apoB100. As will become obvious, apoB100 lipoprotein particles are much more important in atherogenesis than apoB48 lipoprotein particles because the number of apoB100 particles, almost always, is overwhelmingly greater than the number of apoB48 particles. For example, as just noted above, at the peak of the postprandial period, even in patients who are hypertriglyceridemic, with the prominent exception of those with remnant lipoprotein disorder, there are approximately 5 to 10 times more VLDL apoB100 particles than apoB48 particles. Accordingly, for convenience and in accord with usual practice, we will use apoB and apoB100 interchangeably since virtually all the apoB particles present in plasma, with the prominent but unusual exception of remnant lipoprotein disorder, are apoB100 lipoprotein particles.

1.1.2 Anatomy of the ApoB48 and ApoB100 Lipoprotein Particles

The major structural features of the apoB48 and the apoB100 lipoprotein particles are illustrated in Figure 1.1. Each particle has a coat and a core. Most of the lipids within the particle – cholesterol ester and triglyceride – are present within the core and the differences in size of the particles are due to differences in the mass of core lipids. The relative proportion of the core lipids differs and these differences are also characteristic of the different apoB lipoprotein particles.

For the chylomicrons and CR particles, the coat consists of a phospholipid monolayer into which an apoB48 molecule is intercalated, whereas for VLDL, IDL and LDL particles, the coat consists of a phospholipid monolayer into which one apoB100 molecule is intercalated. ApoB48 and apoB100 wrap around the outer phospholipid monolayer of the lipoprotein particles in which they are found and by doing so provide a structural backbone for the particle. Because there is only one apoB48 molecule per particle, the number of chylomicrons and CR is equal to the plasma concentration of apoB48. Similarly, the sum of VLDL, IDL, LDL, and Lp(a) – an LDL particle to which a molecule of apo(a) has been attached – is equal to the plasma apoB100.

Because apoB100 and apoB48 are critical to the architectural structure of the particle, in contrast to the many other apolipoproteins that may be present, or to the core lipids, they are fixed constituents of the particle during its entire lifetime. Free cholesterol has a limited solubility in phospholipid membranes and that is where it is found in the coat of the lipoprotein particles. By contrast, cholesterol ester – that is, cholesterol to which a fatty acid has been joined – is virtually insoluble and immiscible in water and accordingly is found within the core of the particle. This also applies to triglyceride, which is also insoluble and immiscible in water.

Although apoB48 and apoB100 are the signature apolipoproteins, a series of other apolipoproteins including apoE, apoCI, apoCII, apoCIII, apoAI, apoAIV, apoAV are scattered on the surface of chylomicrons and VLDL. Some of these are present when the particle is secreted from its site of synthesis while others are transferred from other lipoprotein particles during their lifetimes in plasma. Many influence critical steps in the metabolism of the lipoprotein particles whereas the function(s) of others remains unknown. In contrast to apoB48 and apoB100, these apolipoproteins are not fixed constituents of the particles but attach and detach relatively freely during their lifetime.

Much remains to be learned about the function of these apolipoproteins. ApoCIII, in particular, seems to be an important determinant of VLDL metabolism and there is considerable evidence linking increased apoCIII to increased cardiovascular risk.[7,8] It remains uncertain, however, whether this association is independent of any effect of apoCIII on VLDL or LDL particle number. Even if it were not, as is not unlikely, that would not diminish the significance of apoCIII as a potential therapeutic tool to manipulate VLDL or LDL particle number.

The major components of apoB48 and apoB100 particles are summarized in *Table 1*.[9]

Table 1.1 Major Components of ApoB48 and ApoB100 Particles

	Chylomicron	VLDL	IDL	LDL
Density (g/ml)	~ 0.93	0.93-1.006	1.006-1.019	1.019-1.063
Diameter (nm)	75-1200	30-80	25-35	18-25
Surface components				
Total Apolipoprotein content	1-2%	8%	19%	22%
ApoB48	+	-	-	-
ApoB100	-	+	+	+
ApoCI	+	+	+	-
ApoCII	+	+	+	-
ApoCIII	+	+	+	-
ApoE	+	+	+	-
ApoAI	+	+	-	-
ApoAIV	+	+	-	-
ApoAV	+	ı	-	-
Surface Lipids				
Cholesterol	1-3%	7%	9%	8%
Phospholipids	7-9%	18%	19%	22%
Core Lipids				
Triglycerides	85-90%	55%	23%	6%
Cholesterol Esters	1 - 3%	12%	29%	42%

1.1.3 The ApoB48 Lipoprotein Particles: Chylomicrons and Chylomicron Remnants

Physiological Role

The triglyceride and cholesterol within the food we eat are absorbed by the microvillar cells of the intestine, within which they are assembled into nascent chylomicron particles, which are secreted into the lymph and then into plasma, and within which they are delivered via the circulation to selected sites within our bodies. The amount of each of these major lipids that we ingest per day varies and is determined by the wealth of the society in which we live, our individual wealth within that society, and the dietary culture of our society. The mass of triglycerides always far exceeds the mass of cholesterol. On average, in affluent Western cultures, we ingest about 100 g of tri-glycerides versus 500 mg or less cholesterol per day. Triglycerides provide us with fatty acids and fatty acids are one of our principal sources of energy (Figure 1.2).

Synthesis and Secretion of ApoB48 Lipoprotein Particles

An overview of the synthesis and metabolism of chylomicrons is presented in *Figure 1.2*. Chylomicron particles are very large particles, 75-1200 nm in diameter, and consist principally of triglycerides (90%) with lesser amounts of phospholipids (approximately 9%), cholesterol (1-3%) and only small amounts of protein (1-2%). Each contains one molecule of apoB48, which stays with the particle during its lifetime. Within the lumen of the small intestine, the dietary triglycerides are hydrolyzed by pancreatic lipases. The fatty acids that are released by pancreatic lipase from the dietary triglyceride as well as the cholesterol that was ingested enter the enterocytes of the small intestine

FIGURE 1.2

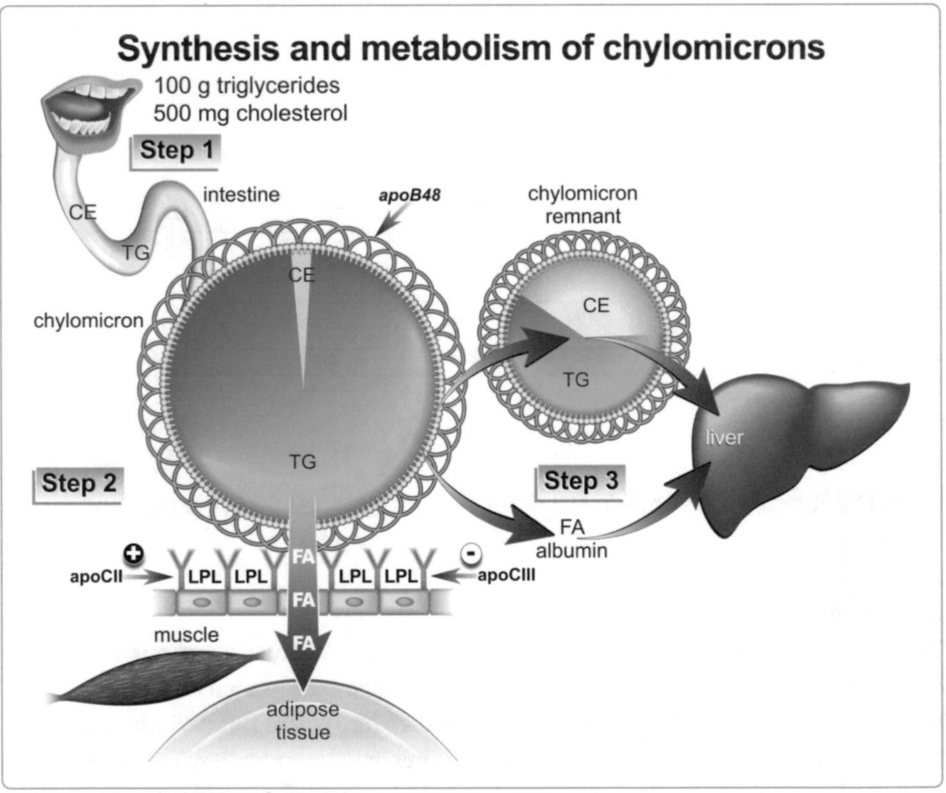

Synthesis and metabolism of chylomicrons

100 g triglycerides
500 mg cholesterol

Step 1

intestine   *apoB48*   chylomicron remnant

CE

TG

chylomicron

CE

CE

TG

liver

TG

Step 2

Step 3

FA
albumin

apoCII → LPL LPL   LPL LPL ← apoCIII

FA

FA

muscle   FA

adipose tissue

and are reformed into triglycerides. Most of the cholesterol that has been absorbed or synthesized within the enterocytes is esterified and the triglycerides and CE are integrated into the core of a nascent chylomicron particle around the surface of which an apoB48 molecule is wrapped.

Step 1: Chylomicrons are secreted by the enterocytes into the intestinal lymphatics and then enter the systemic circulation via the thoracic duct

Within the lymphatics and the systemic circulation, a series of apolipoproteins are added to their surface. These additional apolipoproteins modify the downstream metabolic fate of the chylomicron particle. During fasting, the smallest chylomicron particles continue to be secreted, but at low rates, and these contribute to the small amount of apoB48 that can be detected in fasting plasma.

Step 2: Interaction of Chylomicrons with Adipose Tissue and Skeletal Muscle

Breakdown or hydrolysis of the triglyceride within a chylomicron particle can only occur after it binds to multiple contiguous molecules of lipoprotein lipase (LPL) which, in turn, are bound to the endothelial surface of the capillary endothelium of adipose tissue, and skeletal and cardiac muscle (Figure 1.2). Normally, about 70% of the triglycerides within the core of the chylomicron particle are hydrolyzed by LPL, after the LPL has been activated by apoCII. ApoCII is an apolipoprotein which is present on the surface of the chylomicron particle and which is essential for normal activity of LPL whereas apoCIII, which is also present on the phospholipid monolayer coat of the particle, appears to inhibit LPL activity.

Most of the fatty acids which are released from the chylomicron particle enter the nearby adipocytes or myocytes and are rapidly reformed into triglycerides. However, a significant number bind to albumin and are swept away to enter the systemic circulation. The fraction that goes one way is inversely proportional to the fraction that goes the other. If most of the fatty acids enter the adipocytes – that is, if most are trapped by the adipocyte – few will immediately enter plasma and, accordingly, few will reach the liver. However, if the portion that enters adipocytes is reduced, more will enter plasma and more will reach the liver. This matters for our cardiovascular health because fatty acid flux to the liver is a major determinant of hepatic VLDL secretion which, in turn, is a major determinant of apoB particle number in plasma and therefore of atherogenic risk. Thus, impaired fatty acid trapping by adipose tissue is one of the major physiological causes of elevated apoB or HyperapoB.[10]

By contrast, little or none of the cholesterol ester core of the chylomicron particle is hydrolyzed or sequestered in adipose tissue and therefore remains with the rest of the chylomicron particle. Because so much of the core triglyceride has been broken down, the chylomicron particle is now much smaller and relatively enriched in cholesterol. Moreover, as the particle gets so much smaller, much of the surface phospholipids, which are now in excess, and many of the surface apolipoproteins – but not, of course, apoB48 itself – are detached from the chylomicron particles. The phospholipids of the external monolayer along with the free cholesterol within it become incorporated into high-density lipoprotein (HDL) particles. There is, therefore, a direct relation between the effectiveness with which chylomicrons are metabolized peripherally and the rate at which HDL is synthesized.

Step 3: Uptake of CR by the Liver

These changes in the structure and volume of the chylomicron particle due to LPL are profound and rapid. The result is a CR, a much smaller particle, relatively enriched in cholesterol, which is released from the endothelial surface usually with a number of molecules of LPL still attached. Within only a few minutes, these CR, which are normal products of the metabolism of the chylomicron particles, are removed from the circulation by attaching to the cell membrane of the hepatocyte and then being internalized (Figure 1.2).

The process of binding and internalization of the CR is complex and involves interaction with hepatic lipase, LPL, apoE, and heparin sulfate proteoglycans in addition to receptors, such as the LDL receptor and the LDL-receptor related protein (LRP).[11] Because apoB48 does not contain the binding region to the LDL receptor that is within the full-length apoB100, the LDL pathway cannot be directly involved in removal of CR.

1.1.4 The ApoB100 Lipoproteins Particles: VLDL, IDL, LDL

In this segment, we will follow a VLDL particle from its formation in the liver, through its interaction with LPL and conversion to an IDL particle, and finally to an LDL particle (Figure 1.3). VLDL particles are triglyceride-rich and have a half-life of 3-4 hours whereas LDL particles are cholesterol-rich and have a half-life of 3-4 days. This marked difference in particle survival time explains why there are almost always 9 times more LDL particles than VLDL particles (Figure 1.4). Thus, to repeat, there are two reasons that LDL is a far more important determinant of atherogenic risk than VLDL. First, there are many more LDL particles than VLDL particles and second, LDL particles are smaller and therefore are able to enter the arterial wall more easily than VLDL particles.

FIGURE 1.3

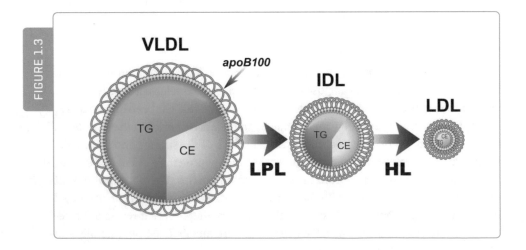

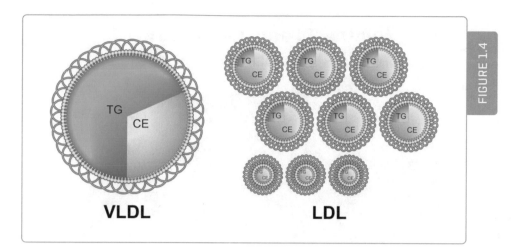

FIGURE 1.4

Step 1: Synthesis and Secretion of VLDL Particles

Much is known about how VLDL particles are constructed within the liver but, at the same time, much remains unknown.[1-5,12-15] In particular, we do not know how the major lipids, triglycerides and cholesterol ester are moved from the sites at which they are made and stored within the hepatocyte to the site(s) at which apoB100 lipoprotein particles are assembled. Moreover, no one knows exactly what regulates the rate at which VLDL particles are secreted by the hepatocyte versus what determines just how much core lipid each contains. A general overview of VLDL metabolism is provided in Figure 1.5.

We do know that apoB100 – the key structural component of VLDL – is synthesized in the rough endoplasmic reticulum (RER) while the principal lipids it will transport from the cell – triglycerides and cholesterol ester – are synthesized in both the rough and smooth endoplasmic reticulum (SER). ApoB100 molecules are synthesized steadily throughout the day. However, only a relatively small number of these newly synthesized apoB molecules successfully associate with lipids and become nascent VLDL particles. Most are hydrolyzed shortly after they are synthesized and it is this step that appears to be the decisive determinant of the rate at which apoB100 lipoprotein particles are secreted by the liver. The early association with lipids is obviously a key step as absence of the protein that transfers cholesterol ester and triglycerides to be associated with nascent VLDL or chylomicron particles – microsomal triglyceride transport protein (MTP) – results in absent secretion of apoB particles from the intestines and the liver.

Other apolipoproteins, such as apoCIII and apoAV, also influence the synthesis and secretion of VLDL particles, perhaps because of effects on triglyceride synthesis and secretion although perhaps also due to an effect on apoB secretion rates. Both apoCIII

FIGURE 1.5

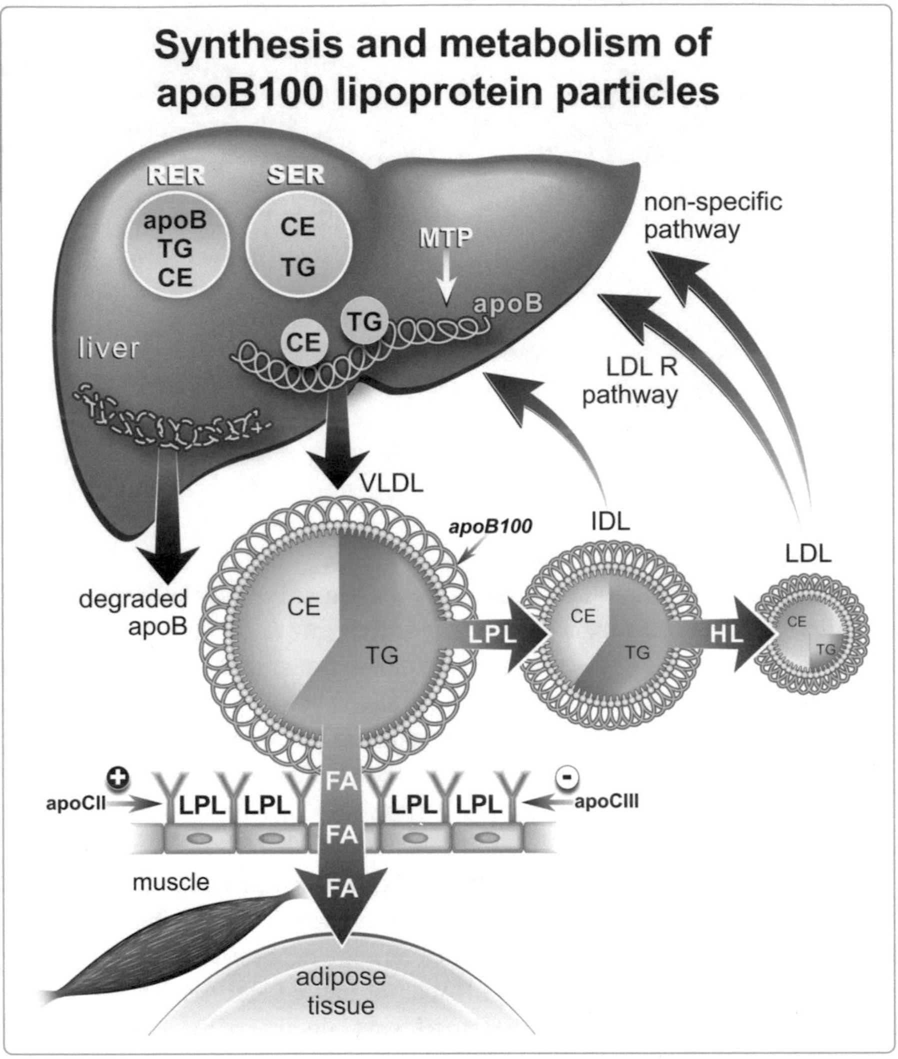

Synthesis and metabolism of apoB100 lipoprotein particles

and apoAV may also interfere with VLDL clearance by diminishing the effectiveness of the interaction of VLDL and LPL.

Because the fraction of apoB molecules that survive to be incorporated in a VLDL particle is variable, the number of VLDL particles secreted into plasma per day can vary substantially. Because VLDL particles are transformed into LDL particles, the number of LDL particles produced per day can vary substantially. Because increased secretion of VLDL particles is the commonest cause of increased LDL particle number in plasma, understanding the determinants of VLDL secretion is of critical importance (Figure 1.5).

The key principles are:

1) The rate at which VLDL particles are secreted can vary substantially and this matters because the rate at which LDL particles are formed is a function of the rate at which VLDL particles are secreted.

2) The amount of triglyceride per VLDL particle can vary substantially. Therefore, the rate at which triglycerides can be removed from the liver is a function of the mass of triglyceride per VLDL particle that is secreted and the number of VLDL particles secreted per unit time.

3) Secretion of VLDL particles is an integral mechanism to maintain cholesterol as well as triglyceride homeostasis within the hepatocyte.

Step 2: Interaction of VLDL with LPL

VLDL transports triglyceride to peripheral tissues, principally adipose tissue and skeletal muscle, where LPL hydrolyzes the triglyceride within VLDL just as LPL hydrolyzes the triglyceride within chylomicrons. There are three reasons why chylomicrons are cleared from the circulation in a few minutes whereas VLDL particles are cleared in a few hours. First, there are many more VLDL particles than chylomicron particles; second, VLDL particles bind less readily to LPL than chylomicrons; and third, chylomicron particles undergo only one interaction in peripheral tissue in which most of their triglyceride is removed whereas VLDL must bind to LPL several times (Figure 1.5).

On the other hand, because there are so many times more VLDL than chylomicron particles (10 times), even though the affinity of VLDL binding to LPL is so much less than chylomicrons (10 times), VLDL as a class can effectively compete for binding to LPL with chylomicrons. This likely explains why fasting levels of triglyceride, which reflects levels of VLDL, are the major predictor of the rate at which chylomicrons are cleared from plasma.[16]

Step 3: Fate of VLDL Particles after Release from Adipose Tissue

After their interactions with adipose tissue, the VLDL particles are now smaller, contain less triglyceride, but are relatively enriched in cholesterol ester and contain fewer apolipoproteins on their surface and may either be removed from the circulation by the liver or converted into IDL (Figure 1.5). IDL contain roughly equal amounts of triglyceride and cholesterol ester in their core and IDL, in turn, are either removed by the liver or converted into LDL particles by virtue of interaction with hepatic lipase. Unfortunately, little is understood as to what determines the fate of VLDL particles, which means that little is understood as to the regulation of the production of LDL particles. In rats and most other species, relatively few VLDL particles are converted to LDL particles. Thus rats, in contrast to man, in whom a relatively large portion of VLDL particles are converted to LDL particles, are resistant to atherogenesis whereas man is susceptible.

Step 4: LDL

LDL particles are the smallest and most numerous of the apoB100 particles. Most of the triglyceride has been removed from the core of the apoB100, which is now made up principally of cholesterol ester. All, or almost all of the apolipoproteins, have been removed from the surface except, of course, the single molecule of apoB100. The great majority of LDL particles – probably more than 90% – are removed from plasma by the liver either by the LDL-receptor pathway or by non-specific pathways (Figure 1.5). The general view is that the number of LDL particles is principally determined by the rate at which they are removed. This is not correct. Increased production of LDL particles is a much more common cause of increased LDL particle number than impaired clearance.[17]

1.1.5 Lipoprotein(a)

A particle of Lp(a) is a hybrid: an LDL particle which has been covalently linked by a disulfide bridge to a molecule of apolipoprotein (a). Apo(a) is a complex molecule, one component of which is a number of cysteine-rich Kringle IV repeats. Because the number of repeats is variable, there is great heterogeneity in isoform size making assays that accurately quantitate Lp(a) molecular mass challenging to develop. Although the strengths of the epidemiological relations have varied over time, there is credible evidence, particularly from Mendelian randomization studies, that increases in Lp(a) are associated with increases in cardiovascular risk.[18,19,20] The evidence that Lp(a) is a causal factor in the pathogenesis of calcific aortic stenosis is, if anything, stronger.[21] There has been much speculation as to how Lp(a) promotes atherogenesis – perhaps by inhibiting fibrinolysis, perhaps by inhibiting plasminogen and perhaps by local effects at the lesion site within the arterial wall. However, before Lp(a) should become a routine test, we believe further work is required on the assays to determine if risk relates to the number of Lp(a) particles or to properties of the (a) molecule such as its length. The distribution of Lp(a) levels within the population is highly skewed and dispute remains as to the level as which risk rises and there should be evidence of benefit from randomized trials of clinical benefit from lowering of Lpa(a). Nicotinic acid is the therapeutic agent of choice at the moment and it was disappointing not to see a positive effect on event rate in the AIM-HIGH clinical trial.[22] These limitations in knowledge and laboratory technique explain why Lp(a) is not in the apoB algorithm. We look forward to this changing.

1.2 Heterogeneity in the ApoB Lipoprotein Particles

> **VLDL heterogeneity**
>
> VLDL particles are the triglyceride-rich lipoproteins secreted by the liver. They differ in size, composition and metabolic fate. If only plasma triglyceride is measured, physicians do not know which VLDL particles are present. However, by combining triglycerides with cholesterol and apoB and applying the apoB diagnostic algorithm, VLDL particles, chylomicron particles, chylomicron remnant particles and VLDL remnants can be differentiated and identified.

> **LDL heterogeneity**
>
> LDL particles are cholesterol-rich lipoproteins, which are generally products of VLDL metabolism. LDL particles differ in size and cholesterol content. All LDL particles are atherogenic although opinions differ whether small cholesterol-depleted LDL are more atherogenic than large cholesterol-enriched LDL particles. Accordingly, LDL-C does not accurately reflect LDL particle number when either cholesterol-enriched or cholesterol-depleted LDL particles are present. Since there are 9 times more LDL than VLDL particles, LDL particle number determines plasma apoB.

1.2.1 Introduction

There are major differences in the composition of VLDL and LDL particles, differences which influence their metabolic fate and their atherogenic risk and therefore differences which should be taken into account for maximal accuracy in diagnosis and greatest benefit from therapy. In this section we will outline how both VLDL and LDL particles can differ in composition and therefore why the concentration of triglycerides and LDL-C do not necessarily equal the number of VLDL and LDL particles respectively.

1.2.2 VLDL Heterogeneity

Conceptually, VLDL particles can be divided into three subclasses: VLDLI (Sf 100-400), VLDLII (Sf 60-100), and VLDLIII (Sf 20-60).[1,23,24] VLDLI are the largest, most triglyceride-rich VLDL particles secreted by the liver whereas VLDLIII are the smallest and contain the most cholesterol ester. VLDLII are intermediate in composition. (*Figure 1.6 part A*) These are normal variants of VLDL composition and their atherogenic risk – one versus another or indeed any at all – is uncertain. An alternate approach distinguishes two subclasses: VLDL1 (Sf 60-400) and VLDL2 (Sf 20-60): VLDL1 encompassing both VLDLI and VLDLII. No matter how much or how little core lipid they contain, each VLDL particle has one apoB100 molecule (Figure 1.6 part A).

VLDL particles are normally hydrolyzed by LPL and the progressive removal of triglyceride produces smaller VLDL particles and ultimately IDL and LDL particles (Figure 1.3 and 1.5). These are all normal particles, present in different numbers in different individuals. The normal metabolic transformation of VLDL particles occurs within a few hours (half-life of 4-6 hours). By contrast, VLDL remnants are abnormal VLDL particles, which are enriched in cholesterol ester compared with other VLDL particles (Figure 1.6 part B). The excess cholesterol is due to the continued exchange of core lipids – cholesterol ester and triglyceride – between VLDL and HDL/LDL particles under circumstances when clearance of VLDL and partially metabolized chylomicron particles is markedly delayed. It is the marked delay that produces the extra time for the marked increase in cholesterol ester in the VLDL and CR to occur.

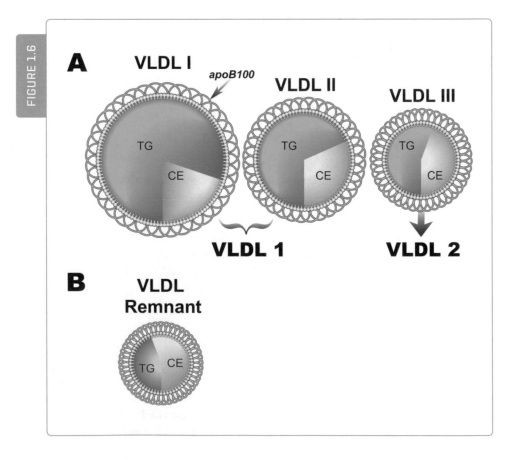

FIGURE 1.6

Remnant lipoprotein disorder, or type III dyslipoproteinemia, is the paradigmatic clinical example of this metabolic abnormality.[25,26] Atherogenic risk in these patients is markedly increased and that is why there is such great concern about remnant lipo-protein particles. However, remnant particle number in these patients is increased at least 20 to 40 fold above that in other circumstances.[27,28] So, in remnant lipoprotein disorder, remnants equal or outnumber normal VLDL particles. How much additional clinical risk there is with remnant particle numbers in the more usual range when remnants are one-fifth or less of the total VLDL particle number remains unknown.

1.2.2.1 VLDL Heterogeneity: Regulation of VLDL Composition and Particle Number

Three different processes interact to account for heterogeneity in the composition of VLDL particles. The first is differences in the composition of the VLDL particles that are secreted. Thus, the mass of triglyceride incorporated into each nascent apoB particle may differ substantially: the more triglyceride that incorporated into a nascent particle, the larger the VLDL particle that will be secreted.[1,23,24,29] The actual mass of triglyceride that is incorporated will be determined by the mass of triglyceride available to be incor-porated in the smooth endoplasmic reticulum or the Golgi versus the number of nascent apoB molecules available to incorporate these masses of triglyceride (Figure 1.5).

If large amounts of triglyceride are incorporated into small numbers of apoB particles, the liver will secrete small numbers of large triglyceride-rich VLDL I particles (Figure 1.7, number 1). However, if large amounts of triglyceride are incorporated into large num-bers of apoB particles, the liver will secrete large numbers of VLDL particles with average amounts of triglyceride (VLDL II) (Figure 1.7, number 2). Increased secretion of relatively triglyceride-poor, cholesterol-rich VLDL particles (VLDL III) (Figure 1.7, number 3) has also been documented in patients with NormoTG HyperapoB, such as patients with familial hypercholesterolemia.[17]

With increased secretion of either VLDL II or VLDL III particles, increased pro-duction of LDL particles will occur and total plasma apoB will be elevated. LDL heterogeneity will be discussed below but VLDL I particles tend to be converted into cholesterol-depleted LDL III particles whereas VLDL III particles tend to be converted into cholesterol-enriched LDL I particles (Figure 1.7).[23,24,30]

The second process that regulates the composition of VLDL particles is progressive hydrolysis of triglyceride by LPL in peripheral tissues as described in paragraph 1.1.4. This results in the sequential conversion of VLDL I into VLDL II into VLDL III particles. It should be noted that a larger proportion of VLDL II and VLDL III particles will be converted into LDL particles than VLDL I particles.[23,24,30]

The third process that influences the composition of VLDL particles is exchange of the core lipids – cholesterol ester and triglyceride – in the plasma compartment. This

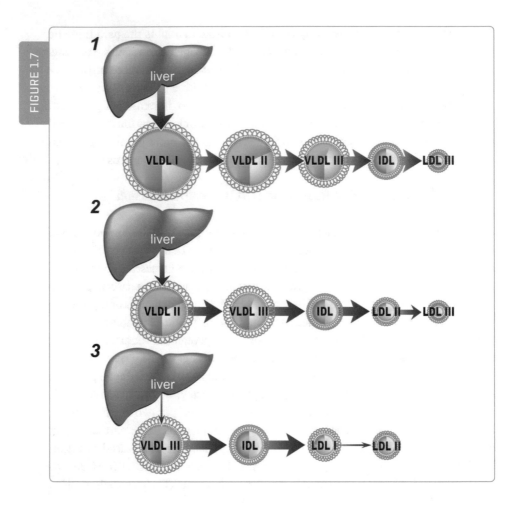

FIGURE 1.7

process, which was alluded to above and will be explained in the section below, results in an increase in cholesterol ester in VLDL particles versus an increase in triglyceride in LDL and HDL particles. Indeed, the majority of cholesterol ester in VLDL probably originates by this process and, as noted above, it is an exaggeration of this process that produces the abnormal remnant particles in remnant lipoprotein disorder.

1.2.2.2 Hypertriglyceridemia due to Excess VLDL

Based on the previous section, it follows that hypertriglyceridemia due to VLDL may be due either to an increased mass of triglycerides within a normal number of VLDL particles or to an increased number of VLDL particles with an average triglyceride content. Because an important proportion of VLDL particles are converted into LDL particles and because the proportion of LDL to VLDL particles is close to constant, the difference in VLDL particle number will result in a marked difference in LDL particle number.

FIGURE 1.8

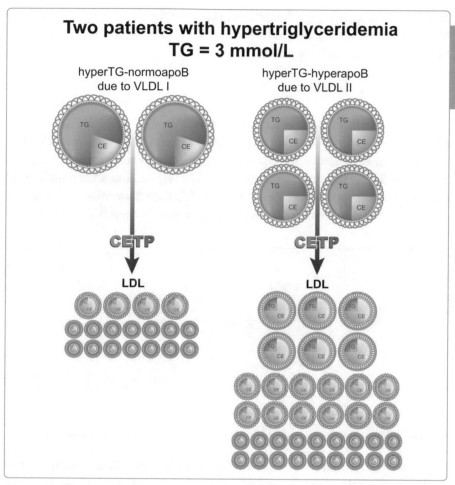

Thus the two hypertriglyceridemic phenotypes due to VLDL are HyperTG NormoapoB and HyperTG HyperapoB (Figure 1.8). Just measuring plasma triglyceride or LDL-C will not distinguish these two, whereas measuring triglyceride, total cholesterol and apoB will.

This is a distinction with a difference – a real and substantial difference – since HyperTG HyperapoB markedly increases vascular risk whereas HyperTG NormoapoB does not.[29,31] The difference in risk relates principally to the difference in LDL particle number between the two phenotypes since in both phenotypes, there are 9 times more LDL particles than VLDL particles. Many have assumed that when apoB is increased in hypertriglyceridemic patients, this is due principally to an increase in VLDL apoB. Despite a few reports to the contrary,[32] the bulk of the literature demonstrates this view to be incorrect.[1,29] VLDL apoB is increased in such patients. However, since there are 9 times more LDL particles, it is the increase in LDL particles that is the principal reason for the increase in total apoB. The increase in the VLDL apoB accounts for only a very small portion of the total increase in apoB.

1.2.3 LDL Heterogeneity

Just as VLDL particles differ in size and composition so do LDL particles.[33,34] LDL particles are often divided into large, cholesterol-rich and small cholesterol-depleted particles but the physiological and pathological realities are more complex than this. To illustrate these, three subclasses are required: LDLI are the largest and most buoyant and contain the most cholesterol ester whereas LDLIII are the smallest, densest, and contain the least cholesterol while LDLII are intermediate in composition (Figure 1.9).

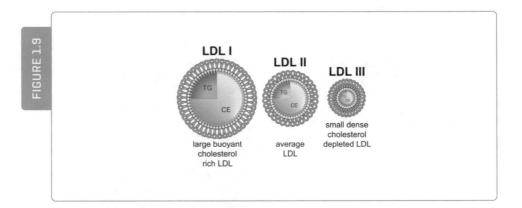

FIGURE 1.9

LDL particles differ in size due to differences in the total mass of lipids in their core and the relative proportions of cholesterol ester and triglyceride in their core. For some time, small dense LDL were felt to be unimportant because they contained less cholesterol than larger LDL particles and delivery of cholesterol to the arterial wall was felt to be the key to atherogenesis. However, an extensive series of experimental and clinical studies suggested small dense LDL particles might be even more atherogenic than their larger counterparts. The reasons for this include their smaller size, the greater ease with which they bind to collagen and elastin within the arterial wall and the more susceptible they are to glycation and oxidation.[1,34,35,36]

Although small cholesterol-depleted LDL particles may be particularly dangerous – the in vitro evidence is impressive – in our view, the best epidemiological evidence at the moment supports the conclusion that all LDL particles are atherogenic and that there is no major difference in the risk they pose. The smaller ones may get in easier, but the larger ones will deposit more cholesterol. There is, as yet, no compelling evidence that LDL composition independent of LDL particle number, influences risk.

This may well represent a limitation in the power of the epidemiological methods and therefore the power of the evidence they produce. Nevertheless, this is where the balance of the evidence lies.

Therefore the number of particles, not their composition, is the primary determinant of risk from LDL. The practical reality is that if only LDL-C is measured in a patient, LDL particle number cannot be inferred. In *Figure 1.10* two patients have an LDL cholesterol of 3 mmol/L. In the patient in the left panel, a higher number of small, cholesterol-depleted LDL particles is present whereas in the patient in the right panel, a smaller number of larger, cholesterol-enriched LDL particles is present. So, in the patient in the left panel, the LDL particle number will be greater than the LDL-C suggests. By contrast, LDL particle number will be less than LDL-C suggests in the patient in the right panel. The net result is that LDL-C will underestimate risk if cholesterol-depleted LDL III particles predominate and overestimate risk if cholesterol-enriched LDL-I particles predominate. Only if an average mass of cholesterol per LDL particle is present will LDL-C equal LDL particle number. Without measuring apoB or LDL particle number, one cannot know which type of LDL and how many LDL particles are present.

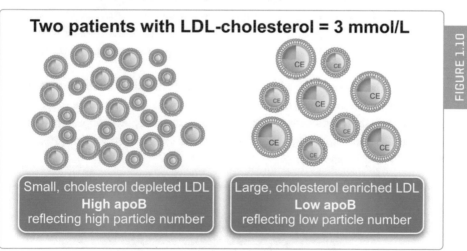

Two patients with LDL-cholesterol = 3 mmol/L

Small, cholesterol depleted LDL
High apoB
reflecting high particle number

Large, cholesterol enriched LDL
Low apoB
reflecting low particle number

FIGURE 1.10

1.2.3.1 The Metabolic Mechanisms Responsible for Cholesterol Composition of LDL Particles

Heterogeneity in the composition of LDL and VLDL particles is the consequence of two different processes, each of which contributes importantly to the final result. First, as described in the section on heterogeneity of VLDL particles, the nature of the VLDL particle that was secreted will influence the nature of the LDL metabolic product. Thus, triglyceride-enriched VLDL I particles disproportionately become cholesterol-depleted LDL III particles whereas triglyceride-depleted cholesterol-enriched VLDL

III particles are disproportionately converted into LDL I particles (Figure 1.7). These tendencies in what type of LDL particle results from what type of VLDL particle reflect differences in the starting composition of the particle. An important difference is also the proportion of VLDL particles that are converted to LDL particles being least with VLDLI and greatest with VLDLIII.

Most attention has focused on the second process that we will now review: the cholesterol ester transfer protein (CETP) mediated core lipid exchanges and transfers.[1,34,35]

Cholesterol ester and triglycerides are both immiscible in water and that is why they are present within the core of the lipoprotein particle, the coat of which is made up of phospholipids and apoB. It is the properties of the coat that allow the particle to be miscible in water and therefore to be able to transport the immiscible core lipids within the water medium that is plasma.

CETP is a hydrophobic glycoprotein, which is synthesized in the liver and which circulates in plasma bound principally to HDL. By forming a bridge between lipoprotein particles, CETP allows molecules of triglyceride and cholesterol ester to be transferred or exchanged amongst them.

Transfer is the process by which one molecule of either triglyceride or cholesterol ester moves from one lipoprotein particle to another in return for which another molecule of the same type moves the other way (Figure 1.11). Since transfer involves the movement of like for like, no net difference in composition of the two particles has occurred.

Exchange is the process by which one molecule of cholesterol ester moves from one particle to the other in return for which one molecule of triglyceride moves in the opposite direction. Exchange changes the composition of both lipoprotein particles: one now contains more triglyceride than before, the other more cholesterol ester than previously (Figure 1.11).

Core Lipid Transfer

CE ⟷ CE

TG ⟷ TG

Core Lipid Exchange

CE ⟷ TG

Which of the two processes – transfer or exchange – predominates is determined by how different the composition of the core lipids of the lipoprotein particles is. Thus, if CETP interacts with LDL and HDL, two cholesterol ester-rich lipoproteins, transfer will predominate whereas if CETP interacts with HDL and VLDL or HDL and chylomicrons, exchange will predominate. In other words, CETP is indifferent as to whether it interacts with cholesterol ester or triglyceride.

CETP mediated core lipid exchanges alter lipoprotein particle composition and can alter particle size. Exchange of cholesterol ester from LDL to VLDL can increase the cholesterol ester content of VLDL particles while exchange of triglyceride from VLDL will produce triglyceride-enriched LDL, which can then be modified to smaller, denser, cholesterol-depleted LDL particles (*Figure 1.12*). This occurs as follows: triglyceride molecules within the particle are hydrolyzed by hepatic lipase and likely also by phos-

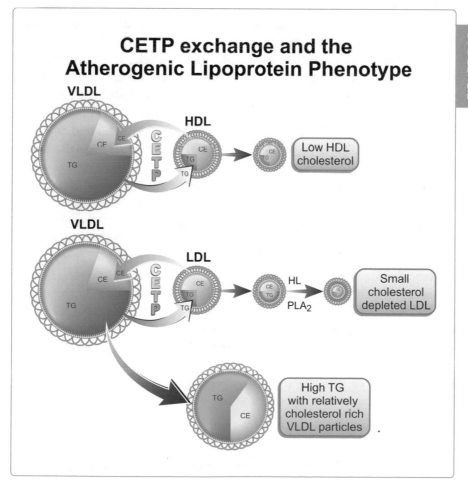

CETP exchange and the Atherogenic Lipoprotein Phenotype

FIGURE 1.12

VLDL · HDL · Low HDL cholesterol

VLDL · LDL · HL · PLA₂ · Small cholesterol depleted LDL

High TG with relatively cholesterol rich VLDL particles

pholipase A2. As they are hydrolyzed, the mass of lipid within the core diminishes and so the particle gets smaller. CETP mediated core lipid exchange increases in the postprandial period and is accelerated by increasing ambient levels of free fatty acids. The same sequence of events likely accounts for the lower HDL-C in hypertriglyceridemic subjects.[37,38] However, HDL-C tends to be lower than the apoA-I particle number. The concept is held widely that triglyceride-rich HDL particles are rapidly cleared and this may be correct relative to normal HDL particles. However, with core lipid exchanges, HDL-C decreases more than apoA-I particle number does. In the event, HDL-C does not begin to reflect HDL particle number any more than LDL-C accurately reflects LDL particle number. Note that VLDL particles become cholesterol enriched in proportion to the degree to which LDL and HDL particles become cholesterol depleted.

1.2.4 The Atherogenic Lipoprotein Phenotype

Gofman and Lindgren[39] were the first to recognize that lipoprotein particles were heterogeneous in size and composition and the first to recognize the clinical implications of these findings. But Gofman's insights and observations were all but lost until Ron Krauss and his colleagues[34,35] provided new and compelling evidence that LDL particles were heterogeneous in composition. They went on to describe the atherogenic lipoprotein phenotype: the combination of hypertriglyceridemia, low HDL-C with predominantly, cholesterol-depleted, LDL particles (Figure 1.12). Multiple studies demonstrated this phenotype to be common in the high-risk states for cardiovascular disease such as diabetes, abdominal obesity, male gender, and postmenopausal women.

The atherogenic lipoprotein phenotype (ALP) is the consequence of the core lipid exchanges just illustrated in Figure 1.12. The emphasis is on the predominance of the small dense LDL particles and there is considerable *in vitro* evidence that the smaller particles may be more atherogenic than larger more cholesterol-enriched LDL particles: they penetrate the arterial wall more easily, they bind to the glycosaminoglycans of the subintimal space more easily and they oxidize more easily. However, as will be reviewed in *Chapter* 5 the more recent epidemiological evidence does not support this conclusion. In our view, the critical limitation of the concept of the ALP is that it does not include particle number. Two individuals with the ALP are illustrated in Figure 1.8. One has a normal VLDL and LDL particle number, the other an increased LDL particle number. As we will demonstrate later, it is the individual with the elevated particle number that is at particularly elevated risk. The number of atherogenic apoB particles is what counts: number trumps composition.

1.3 The Fatty Acid Cycle and the ApoB Lipoprotein Particles

- Total delivery of fatty acids (FA) to the liver is a major determinant of the number/composition of VLDL particles secreted by the liver and therefore a major determinant of LDL particle number in plasma.
- Plasma FA concentration is determined by: 1] the release of FA from adipose tissue and 2] the release of FA from triglyceride-rich lipoproteins by action of LPL.
- Adipose tissue takes up FA from the triglyceride-rich lipoproteins – chylomicrons and VLDL – and converts the FA into triglyceride. This process, FA trapping, is regulated by LPL and by the rate at which adipocytes can synthesize triglyceride.
- The more effective FA trapping is, the less the flux of FA to the liver, either as triglycerides within the chylomicron and VLDL remnant particles, prematurely released from the endothelial surface, or as FA bound to albumin.
- Adipocyte FA trapping is determined by their size and location. Larger adipocytes have greater FA fluxes and release more cytokines and are therefore more atherogenic than smaller adipocytes. Visceral and deep subcutaneous adipose tissue have greater transmembrane FA fluxes and release more cytokines and are therefore more atherogenic than superficial subcutaneous adipose tissue.

1.3.1 Introduction

Fatty acids (FA) are not on tip of everyone's tongue. But they should be. Cholesterol is the word that everyone knows, in part, because it is the 'athero' in atherosclerosis and, in part, because it is the word we use more than any other to relate lipids to vascular disease. FA, in the form of triglycerides, constitute our adipose tissues, which make up the normal thermal and mechanical blanket between our environment and us. That is good but too much of a good thing – or at least too much of a good thing in the wrong place – is no longer good. Excess adipose tissue, as in abdominal obesity, increases our risk of cardiovascular disease in multiple ways.

Amongst these are the fact that FA are such key drivers of the number and composition of VLDL particles secreted by the liver and therefore, such a major determinant of LDL particle number in plasma and therefore of atherogenic risk.[40-42] Furthermore, FA are a major stimulus of intrahepatic cholesterol synthesis.[42] Accordingly, serum cholesterol generally relates more closely to FA intake and metabolism than to cholesterol intake and metabolism.

In this section, we will describe the role of apoB48 and apoB100 lipoproteins as carriers of FA to adipose tissue and the liver and integrate these pathways within the overall cycle of FA flux within the body.

1.3.2 FA Flux and the Adipocyte – the Role of ApoB48 and ApoB100 Lipoproteins

Triglycerides are the storage form of FA and adipose tissue is the only tissue with a substantial capacity to store FA. Indeed, as too many of us have discovered to our sorrow, adipose tissue has an unlimited capacity to expand to store FA. Because other tissues have only a very limited capacity to increase their intracellular triglyceride stores (the liver, unfortunately for the hepatocyte, being a modest exception), FA that are not used by muscle or other tissues must wind up in adipose tissue. Thus, if we are in a positive energy balance, adipose tissue mass will expand whereas, if the reverse is the case, it will recede. The complicating feature that is too often overlooked is that if adipose tissue development is stimulated – say by insulin – FA that are ingested will be sequestered in adipocytes, whose primary metabolic function is to take up and store FA from plasma, and will not be available to myocytes. FA that should have been delivered to muscle and oxidized will be diverted and stored. The consequence will be that energy intake must increase to meet metabolic demands.

Thus, there are three determinants of energy balance, not two: the drive to take in energy, the utilization of energy and the sequestration of energy. Indeed, inappropriate sequestration of energy with the low fat but high carbohydrate diets that have been recommended for so long and so strongly by guideline groups may be major drivers of the increase in abdominal obesity and type 2 diabetes mellitus that have occurred in the past few decades. Inappropriate sequestration of energy will lead, secondarily, to excess caloric intake.

1.3.2.1 Plasma FA and FA Metabolism in Adipose Tissue

FA in plasma originate from adipose tissue or from triglyceride-rich apoB lipoprotein. FA are important energy sources for muscle and liver and other organs (Figure 1.13). Direct uptake from the plasma FA pool is the most obvious route by which FA enter adipocytes, but it is not the most important. That honor goes to FA that enter from the triglyceride-rich lipoproteins, chylomicrons and VLDL.[43] Normally about 70% of the triglyceride is removed from a chylomicron particle once it attaches to a group of LPL molecules on the endothelial surface. The much smaller, triglyceride-depleted particle, called a CR, is released from the endothelial surface and is rapidly taken up by the liver (Figure 1.14A). If the particle were to be released prematurely from the endothelial surface, its triglyceride content would be much greater and the net amount of FA delivered to the liver – by this triglyceride-rich CR – would be correspondingly greater as well (Figure 1.14B).[10] VLDL particles remove excess triglycerides from the liver and, just as chylomicrons do, deliver triglycerides to adipocytes and myocytes. In contrast to chylomicrons, VLDL particles attach and detach multiple times during the metabolic conversion from VLDL particles to LDL particles.

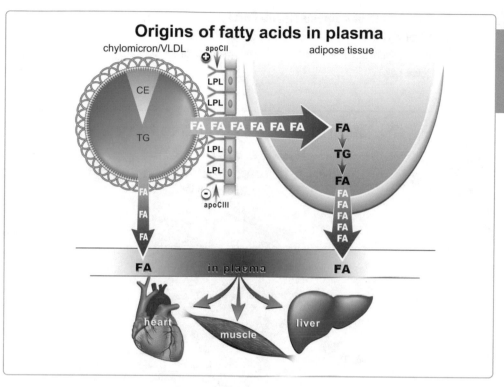

Origins of fatty acids in plasma

FIGURE 1.13

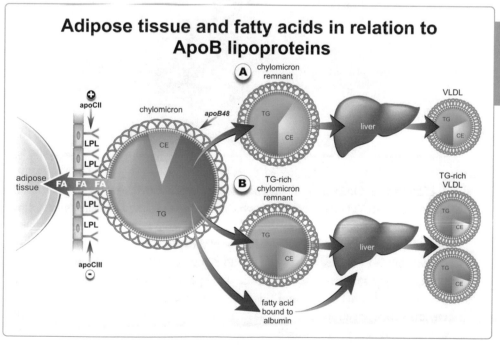

Adipose tissue and fatty acids in relation to ApoB lipoproteins

FIGURE 1.14

Determinants of Adipose Tissue Fatty Acid Uptake from ApoB48 and ApoB100 Triglyceride-Rich Lipoproteins

The key players in the uptake and storage process of FA with adipocytes are illustrated in Figure 1.15

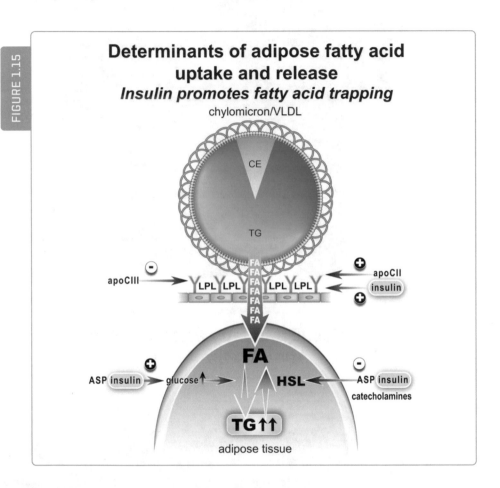

FIGURE 1.15

Determinants of adipose fatty acid uptake and release
Insulin promotes fatty acid trapping

1. **Lipoprotein Lipase:** LPL is the enzyme that hydrolyzes the triglyceride within the chylomicron or VLDL particle. LPL is synthesized and secreted by adipocytes, following which molecules of LPL pass through the endothelial cells and become attached to glycosaminoglycans on the capillary surface of the endothelial cells. Each chylomicron particle binds to between 30 to 40 LPL molecules. ApoCII is a small apolipoprotein present on the surface of the triglyceride-rich lipoprotein particles and is essential for LPL activity. If either LPL or apoCII is absent due to a genetic error in their synthesis, chylomicrons accumulate in the plasma, producing massive hypertriglyceridemia and a high risk of pancreatitis.[44]

2. Insulin: Insulin has many effects that increase FA trapping by adipocytes (*Figure* 1.15).[45-47] Insulin causes more LPL to be released from adipocytes, more LPL to be translocated through the endothelial cell, and subsequently more LPL to appear on the capillary side of the endothelial surface. Insulin also causes increased glucose uptake into adipocytes and therefore increased glycerol-3-phosphate formation. More FA can be joined to glycerol to form triglyceride and therefore FA uptake into the adipocytes increases. By increasing FA uptake into the adipocyte, extracellular FA concentrations are reduced, product inhibition of LPL removed, and lipoprotein triglyceride hydrolysis accelerated. Insulin also inhibits hormone sensitive lipase (HSL), the enzyme that hydrolyzes intracellular triglyceride, thereby reducing the rate at which FA enter the circulation. Thus insulin modulates the effectiveness of FA trapping both during the postprandial period and during fasting. Insulin is most active in the early to mid-postprandial period, consistent with the early elevation and then the rapid decline in plasma insulin levels that occurs after eating.

3. Acylation Stimulating Protein (ASP): ASP is the other peptide which has been shown to regulate FA trapping by adipocytes (*Figure* 1.15). Both insulin and ASP cause triglyceride synthesis to increase within adipocytes.[43] Just like insulin, ASP causes glucose entry to increase within adipocytes by increasing the translocation of glucose transporters from the cytosol to the cell membrane and as a consequence, synthesis of glycerol-3-phosphate increases. Availability of this backbone is a key determinant of the maximal rate of triglyceride synthesis. Also, ASP appears to increase the activity of diacylglycerol acyltransferase, the last enzyme involved in the synthesis of a triglyceride molecule. Both actions promote intracellular triglyceride synthesis and therefore act to increase FA uptake into the adipocyte.[48,49]

ASP also inhibits HSL activity, although not to the same extent as insulin.[43,48,49] However, by increasing re-esterification of the FA liberated by HSL, ASP can reduce the rate at which they leave the adipocyte. Indeed in vitro studies have shown that ASP and insulin together can virtually halt the exit of FA from adipocytes that were maximally stimulated by catecholamines.

1.3.2.2 Release of Fatty Acids from Adipocytes
HSL hydrolyzes intracellular triglyceride to release FA, a portion of which will be re-esterified, but most of which will exit the cell along with the glycerol backbone to which the FA had been attached. HSL activity – and therefore, FA release – is regulated by insulin, catecholamines, and ASP (*Figure* 1.15).[50] HSL comes into play in the first 2-3 hours after a meal, when plasma FA concentrations drop dramatically after which they gradually return to premeal levels, paralleling the changes in plasma insulin. With fasting, basal FA release from adipocytes is greater due to greater HSL activity. Surges of FA release will occur if catecholamines stimulate HSL activity.

1.3.2.3 Consequences of Incomplete FA Trapping by Adipose Tissue

If FA cannot be incorporated into adipose tissue triglyceride stores as rapidly as necessary, LPL will be inhibited by their buildup, triglyceride hydrolysis will stop, and there will be premature detachment of only partially metabolized CR particles. These particles, which will contain more triglyceride than normal, will be taken up by the liver with the result that FA delivery to the liver will increase (Figure 1.14).[10,51]

The second mechanism to increase delivery of FA to the liver results from the FA released by LPL from the triglyceride-rich lipoproteins, which are not taken up by adipocytes, but rather are released into the systemic circulation and bound to albumin. That is, the trapping of FA by adipose tissue is incomplete. FA that were released from triglyceride-rich lipoproteins and taken up in the postprandial period may be released in large amounts from these cells in the period between meals. Indeed, this may be one of the major differences in the metabolism of abdominal adipocytes from lower body adipocytes. The net result in both cases will be increased delivery of FA to the liver bound to albumin (Figure 1.14).[52]

1.3.2.4 Adipocyte Size and Adipose Tissue Location

All adipose tissue is not the same – far from it. Size and location are both critical determinants of adipocyte function.[53,54]

Adipocyte Size

As adipocytes get larger, transmembrane FA flux increases (Figure 1.16). That is, larger adipocytes have greater release of FA and greater triglyceride hydrolysis.[55,56] At the same time, they also have greater uptake of FA and triglyceride synthesis. At steady state, by definition, the total internal and external fluxes of FA are in balance. Even when not in steady state, when the adipocyte is either gaining or losing net triglyceride mass, the difference between intake and output of FA over any day will be small relative to flux in

FIGURE 1.16

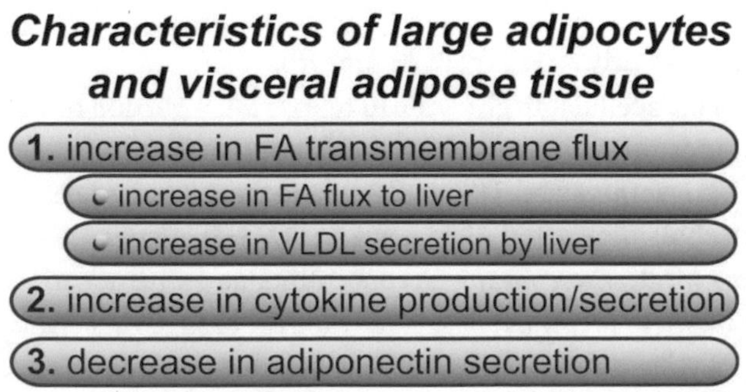

Characteristics of large adipocytes and visceral adipose tissue

1. increase in FA transmembrane flux
   - increase in FA flux to liver
   - increase in VLDL secretion by liver
2. increase in cytokine production/secretion
3. decrease in adiponectin secretion

either direction. Thus, FA transmembrane traffic is a positive function of adipocyte size.[53] Although FA input and output will be in balance, or close to it by the end of the day, they differ in timing during the day. Input of FA predominantly occurs in the postprandial state whereas output is mainly during fasting. As FA are released in greater amounts into the circulation, FA flux to the liver will necessarily increase as well. Therefore, larger adipocytes will lead to increased secretion of VLDL particles by the liver. Cytokine secretion also relates to adipocyte size. Adiponectin secretion, a cytokine associated with beneficial metabolic effects, decreases as adipocyte size increases. By contrast, secretion of tumor necrosis factor-α, a cytokine with adverse metabolic effects, increases. From both perspectives, as a general rule, larger adipocytes are more atherogenic than smaller ones.

Adipocyte Location

But there is a second, likely more important determinant of adipocyte function: adipocyte location. There are three different adipose tissue compartments (Figure 1.17): the superficial and deep subcutaneous adipose tissue and the visceral adipose tissue.[57] The visceral adipose tissue or the upper body adipocytes have the greatest FA fluxes. Thus, they account for more of the removal of FA from triglyceride-rich lipoproteins and also, as we have just pointed out, for more of the addition of FA to plasma. Visceral adipocytes have captured much attention and no doubt the risk of dyslipidemia and dysglycemia increase as visceral adipose tissue mass increases. However, the issue is more interesting.

The superficial subcutaneous adipose tissue is present just under the skin in the arms, legs, and trunk. It acts as a thermal blanket as well as protection against trauma. This is the most organized of the adipose tissue depots with very well demarcated lobules. It is also the most stable metabolically. Once formed, there is a very slow turnover of triglycerides within it. It is also the least well vascularized and the least important for

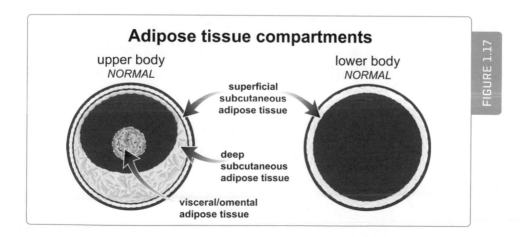

FIGURE 1.17

day-to-day triglyceride clearance from plasma. This zone is the primary long-term storage compartment of FA and we believe the first from a physiological perspective to undergo expansion under circumstances of energy excess. Most of the adipose tissue in the lower limb is made up of superficial subcutaneous adipocytes (Figure 1.17).[54,58]

Adipocytes can enlarge, but only to a certain degree. Then, they proliferate, but little is known of the determinants of whether and how much they do divide.[59] Because the triglyceride formed within the superficial subcutaneous adipocyte zone is so stable, there is little transmembrane flux of FA per day. Therefore, it has little metabolic impact on other tissues such as the liver and striated muscle.

However, once the storage capacity of this primary reservoir is saturated, two other options exist to store excess triglyceride. The first is the deep subcutaneous adipose tissue compartment, which is present principally in the upper body and is separated by a fascial plane from the superficial subcutaneous adipose tissue compartment. Deep subcutaneous adipose tissue is less well organized and its lobules are less well demarcated and more vascular than the superficial subcutaneous adipose tissue. Visceral or omental adipose tissue is the third compartment and it is present only in the abdomen. Here the lobules are the least well developed and the most vascular.

Vascularity in the three adipose tissue compartments differs substantially. It is greatest in omental and least in gluteal. Vascularity is a good index of the metabolic activity of the zone. The more vascularized adipose tissue compartments clear greater amounts of triglycerides in the postprandial period with correspondingly greater uptake of FA (Figure 1.18). During the period between meals, the reverse occurs in that the more active zones release greater amounts of FA from the adipocytes into the systemic circulation. Thus, expansion of the deep subcutaneous adipose tissue and visceral adipose tissue compartments is associated with increased systemic FA flux and the complications that ensue as in consequence.

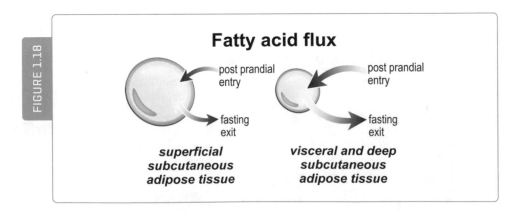

FIGURE 1.18

Fatty acid flux

post prandial entry

fasting exit

superficial subcutaneous adipose tissue

post prandial entry

fasting exit

visceral and deep subcutaneous adipose tissue

1.3.3 Fatty Acid Flux in Hepatocytes

FA can enter hepatocytes either directly as FA from the plasma pool or as triglyceride within the apoB48 remnant chylomicron and as VLDL/IDL particles that are taken up by the liver (Figure 1.19). The mass of FA taken up by the liver relates directly to the FA concentration in plasma. The liver is one of the largest organs in the body, involved in an incredibly broad range of metabolic functions, and accordingly receives a large dual blood supply via the hepatic artery and the portal vein. The liver, therefore, is automatically one of the most important recipients of the FA liberated from adipose tissue.

The FA that reach the liver can be: 1) oxidized completely; 2) converted into ketone bodies; 3) incorporated into structural molecules such as phospholipids; or 4) con-

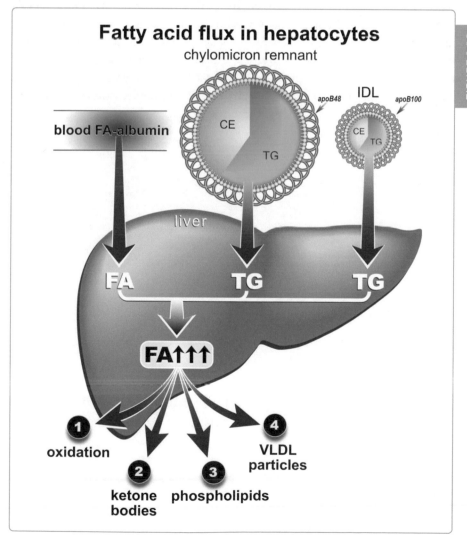

FIGURE 1.19

verted and stored as triglycerides within the cytoplasmic pool, and this is the fate most relevant for us now since the cytosolic triglyceride pool supplies the FA which are secreted within VLDL particles.[60]

The rate at which FA are directly metabolized by oxidation is important because reducing FA oxidation results in increased FA esterification – that is, increased triglyceride synthesis. Thus, by this route, hepatic glucose influences FA partitioning within the liver. The rate of hepatocyte triglyceride synthesis is also directly related to FA delivery to the liver and inversely related to sensitivity to insulin and is therefore increased in insulin resistance. These features are well known and well appreciated. Not well known or well appreciated is the fact that increased delivery of FA to the liver also increases the synthesis of cholesterol ester by virtue of the Acyl-CoA cholesterol acyltransferase (ACAT) reaction (Figure 1.20).[61] ACAT is situated at or very near the endoplasmic reticulum and synthesis of cholesterol ester in this instance results in removal of a cholesterol molecule from the endoplasmic reticulum, which has to be replaced to maintain the functional capacities of the endoplasmic reticulum membrane. Cholesterol synthesis increases in order to do so and indeed there is evidence that this is one of the most important drivers of cholesterol synthesis within the liver. This is a key linkage between FA and cholesterol metabolism. It may also be a key determinant of the number versus the size of VLDL particles that are secreted.

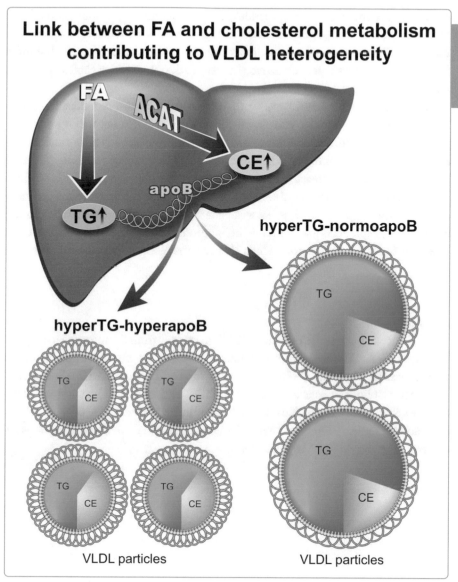

FIGURE 1.20

Link between FA and cholesterol metabolism contributing to VLDL heterogeneity

FA

ACAT

CE↑

apoB

TG↑

hyperTG-normoapoB

TG

CE

hyperTG-hyperapoB

TG   CE

TG   CE

TG   CE

TG   CE

TG

CE

VLDL particles

VLDL particles

1.3.3.1 Regulation of VLDL Secretion by the Liver

VLDL particles remove excess triglyceride from the liver and therefore play a key role in triglyceride homeostasis in the liver. What everyone does not know is that VLDL particles also play a key role in maintaining cholesterol homeostasis in the liver because far more cholesterol reaches the liver than can be broken down into bile acids and secreted.[17,62] The difference is secreted in VLDL particles or transferred to nascent HDL particles. In terms of mass, triglycerides are certainly the major lipid within VLDL particles. The liver can vary the rate at which VLDL particles are secreted and their size. The determinants of the size and number of VLDL particles are unknown but there is evidence suggesting that it relates more directly to the rate at which cholesterol esters are formed than to the mass of triglycerides.

This is a key point (*Figures 1.8 and 1.20*). Secretion of a normal number of triglyceride-enriched VLDL particles will elevate plasma triglycerides but will not increase plasma apoB concentrations because the LDL particle number will be normal. Secretion of an increased number of VLDL particles will also increase plasma triglyceride but, in this case, will increase plasma apoB because the increased secretion of VLDL particles will lead to the increased secretion of LDL particles. The first scenario produces HyperTG NormoapoB, which is not associated with marked increase in cardiovascular risk – except, of course, for remnant lipoprotein disorder – whereas the second produces HyperTG HyperapoB, which is associated with increased cardiovascular risk.

Summary

There is not one but a series of cycles of FA flux, initially from the intestine to adipose tissue, muscle and the liver within chylomicron triglycerides, then from adipose tissue to muscle as FA and to the liver as FA and CR and VLDL particles and finally from the liver back to adipose tissue and muscle as VLDL triglycerides. The back and forth complex character of the traffic is a function of the fact that adipose tissue can both store and later release FA: what comes in can go out again from adipose tissue as FA and from the liver as VLDL triglycerides.

1.4 The Hepatic Cholesterol Cycle and Regulation of ApoB Lipoprotein Particles

- 500 mg of cholesterol per day is synthesized by enterocytes and hepatocytes and we ingest 500 mg of dietary cholesterol per day.
- Free cholesterol is an essential component of all biological membranes to maintain membrane fluidity and function and therefore cell integrity and survival.
- The liver can accumulate cholesterol by multiple routes: 1. Diet or exogenous cholesterol; 2. Re-uptake of endogenous cholesterol from the apoB100 lipoproteins and HDL; 3. De novo synthesis of cholesterol.
- Cholesterol efflux from the liver can take place via: 1. bile acids; 2. secretion/production of apoB lipoproteins; 3. via HDL.
- Increased cholesterol ester within the hepatocyte will result in an increased proportion of newly synthesized apoB molecules being secreted as VLDL apoB lipoprotein particles. This results in increased formation of LDL particles and so plasma apoB will increase.
- LDL particles are irreversibly cleared from plasma either by the LDL-receptor pathway or by alternative nonspecific scavenger pathways. If clearance through the LDL receptor decreases, clearance through the non-specific pathway will increase, but the cost will be a much higher concentration of plasma apoB particles.

1.4.1 Introduction

Cholesterol is vital for life. Without the proper concentration of cholesterol, the membranes around and within our cells would not function and we would die. That being the case, not surprisingly, all cells can make all the cholesterol they need but, somewhat surprisingly, only hepatocytes can break cholesterol down or secrete it from the body in any significant amounts. This almost certainly explains why the liver is at the crossroads of all the major fluxes of cholesterol in the body and means that what happens in the liver determines the level of LDL in plasma and the total mass of cholesterol within the body. Accordingly, in this section, we will review the movements of cholesterol into and out of the liver and try to demonstrate how the liver determines the level of LDL in plasma both by production and removal of LDL particles.

The conventional view is that the level of LDL in plasma is determined by the rate at which LDL particles are cleared from plasma by the LDL pathway, a view supported by masses of seemingly unchallengeable evidence. That said, we believe this view is incomplete and that it expresses only part of the reality that actually exists: namely, that the rate at which LDL particles are produced is the other major determinant of their number in plasma and that the rate at which LDL particles are produced is a function of the rate at which VLDL particles and/or LDL particles are secreted by the liver. Our view springs from, and is anchored in, our perception of the physiological role of the apoB lipoproteins: that their purpose is to secrete excess cholesterol as well as triglyceride from the liver.

The liver is the central tissue for cholesterol homeostasis in the body, the tissue at which all the major fluxes of cholesterol collide, and the endoplasmic reticulum membrane is the central site at which cholesterol homeostasis in the hepatocyte must be maintained. These inward fluxes of cholesterol far exceed the capacity of the hepatocyte to metabolize and secrete cholesterol from the body and therefore, this is where and why apoB plays a major physiological role in the regulation of cholesterol balance within the hepatocyte.[17,62]

1.4.2 Total Body Cholesterol Balance

Of the 500 mg of cholesterol we synthesize per day, most is made in enterocytes and hepatocytes. What we eat contributes about another 500 mg per day and therefore, give or take, a total of about a gram a day of cholesterol is added to the body per day (Figure 1.21). To avoid accumulating cholesterol, the same amount must be lost from

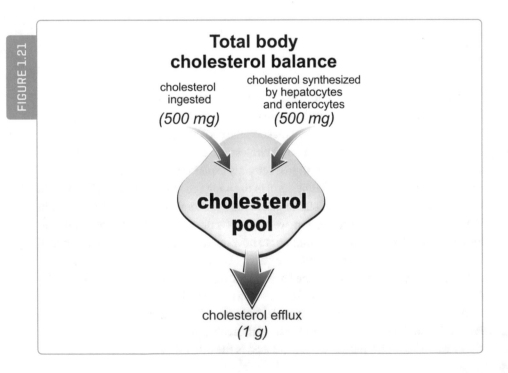

FIGURE 1.21

the body per day but the options to achieve this are limited. Hepatocytes are the only cells that can export cholesterol from the body in any significant quantity and do so: a) by producing bile acids, the breakdown products of cholesterol, and b) by secreting cholesterol directly in bile (Figure 1.22). However, this output is partially offset by the fact that a portion of this cholesterol and bile acids are reabsorbed from the small intestines creating an enterohepatic recycling of cholesterol and bile acids. Nevertheless, in total, about a gram of cholesterol is lost from the body per day via these routes, just enough to balance that which is ingested plus that synthesized.

1.4.2.1 Hepatic Cholesterol Balance

The liver must achieve a steady-state equilibrium in which the amount of cholesterol coming into the liver plus the amount synthesized in the liver equals the amount of cholesterol that leaves the liver. Effluxes must equal influxes. These are the processes we will now review.

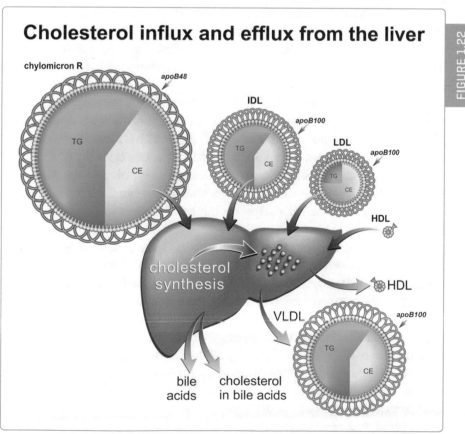

Cholesterol influx and efflux from the liver

FIGURE 1.22

chylomicron R

apoB48

IDL

apoB100

LDL

apoB100

TG

CE

TG

CE

TG

CE

HDL

cholesterol synthesis

HDL

VLDL

apoB100

TG

CE

bile acids

cholesterol in bile acids

1.4.2.2 Cholesterol Influxes to the Hepatocyte

First is the dietary cholesterol (approximately 500 mg/day) plus the cholesterol synthesized in the intestines, both of which are delivered to the liver via chylomicron remnants. *De novo synthesis* of cholesterol within the liver also contributes to positive cholesterol balance. Together, this amounts to approximately 1 gram per day and this alone equals the mass of cholesterol lost from the body per day from the liver. Appreciate also that the mass of dietary cholesterol delivered to the liver is unpredictable and unregulated. However much we choose to eat and at whatever times we choose to eat it, the cholesterol we eat will be delivered, needed or not, to the hepatocyte by chylomicron remnant particles.

However, cholesterol is also returned to the liver by uptake of VLDL, IDL, LDL apoB100 particles as well as HDL particles (Figure 1.22). All contain substantial amounts of cholesterol and so all represent important additional routes of delivery of cholesterol to the liver. For example, in a man with an LDL-C of 2.6 mmol/l and a normal clearance of LDL particles, this would amount to an additional 1.6 g of LDL cholesterol per day.[17] Thus, even in normals, more cholesterol is returned to the liver in LDL particles than leaves it in the bile. But this is only part of the total. The details of the uptake of VLDL particles by the liver are far from clear whereas so much is known about the mechanisms responsible for the uptake of LDL particles. If the results of the stable isotope studies are reliable then another 3 to 4 g of cholesterol would be delivered to the liver by this route.

The liver removes 90% or more of the LDL particles that are formed per day and the rate at which this occurs is one of the two major determinants of the concentration of LDL particles in plasma, the other being the rate at which LDL particles are formed. LDL particles are removed from plasma by two routes. One is via the LDL-receptor pathway, a high-affinity but low-capacity uptake pathway, whereas the other is via multiple routes of non-specific pathways, which are low-affinity but unlimited capacity.[63] How the characteristics of these pathways affect plasma LDL will be detailed below.

HDL also provides an important, albeit complex, route of delivery of cholesterol back to the liver as well as from it. HDL delivers cholesterol directly to the liver either within HDL particles that are taken up by the liver or by transferring cholesterol ester from HDL particles to hepatocytes. In addition, substantial amounts of cholesterol ester are transferred to VLDL and LDL from HDL particles due to the action of CETP (Figure 1.12). Thus, in humans and other species with CETP, LDL turns out to be a major route of delivery of cholesterol from the periphery to the liver.[64,65]

There is no evidence the LDL pathway fulfills any physiologically essential role. All cells can synthesize all the cholesterol they need. Patients who cannot synthesize any apoB particles do just as well from the perspective of cellular cholesterol balance as the rest of us who can. Man stands out as one of the few species (pigs are another) who convert a large portion of the VLDL particles to LDL particles rather than remove them as normal VLDL remnants from plasma and it is only these few species that stand at any risk of developing atherosclerosis. In this regard, we humans appear to be the evolutionary inferiors of so many of our compatriot species.

1.4.2.3 Efflux of Cholesterol from the Liver

As we have seen, the multiple intakes of cholesterol far exceed the limited capacity of the liver to secrete cholesterol dissolved within the bile or as bile acids. But balance must be achieved. Two other routes maintain cholesterol homeostasis, but these have been much less well appreciated, perhaps because they seem counterintuitive within the conventional model of cholesterol transport. The first is within VLDL particles (and occasionally in LDL particles) and the second, curiously enough, is within HDL particles (Figure 1.22). HDL precursor particles can remove cholesterol from hepatocytes just as effectively as from peripheral tissues if not more so and there is evidence of a reciprocal relation between this route and the other that we are now going to focus on: the role of the apoB lipoproteins in maintaining hepatic cholesterol homeostasis.[66,67]

The fate of the cholesterol that enters the liver within lipoprotein particles depends on which lipoprotein particle carries it in (Figure 1.23).[62] The cholesterol that enters within chylomicron particles results in suppression of cholesterol synthesis and decreased synthesis of LDL receptors. However, the cholesterol that enters within LDL particles produces much less suppression of cholesterol and LDL-receptor synthesis. Rather, most of the cholesterol that is released from the LDL lysosome is rapidly esterified by acyl-cholesterol acyltransferase and secreted from the liver within newly synthesized apoB particles. This creates a shunt pathway for cholesterol, which enters the liver within LDL particles and which leaves it within VLDL particles without ever entering the regulatory pool of cholesterol within the liver and therefore without any inhibitory effect on the synthesis of cholesterol and LDL receptors by the hepatocyte. The net result is that cholesterol balance within the hepatocyte is maintained at the cost of increased VLDL secretion and therefore increased apoB, and therefore increased hazard to our arteries (Figure 1.23).

1.4.3 Regulation of Cholesterol Homeostasis in the Liver

The conventional view is that production of cholesterol within the hepatocyte is inversely related to the cholesterol synthesized plus the cholesterol that enters via the LDL pathway. Homeostasis is a simple teeter totter model: action, reaction, balance. That is how things work in the fibroblast in vitro. But that is not how it works in the liver where there appear to be multiple channels of cholesterol, each tracing a somewhat different route within and through the cell, each fulfilling a specific metabolic purpose (*Figure 1.23*). Cholesterol from chylomicrons rapidly enters the regulatory pool with inhibition of cholesterol and LDL-receptor synthesis. Cholesterol from LDL is rapidly esterified and secreted within apoB particles.[62] HDL particles are taken up by the SR-BI receptor, the cholesterol ester hydrolyzed by hepatic cholesterol esterase, and the cholesterol that is released preferentially secreted in the bile.[68-70]

FIGURE 1.23

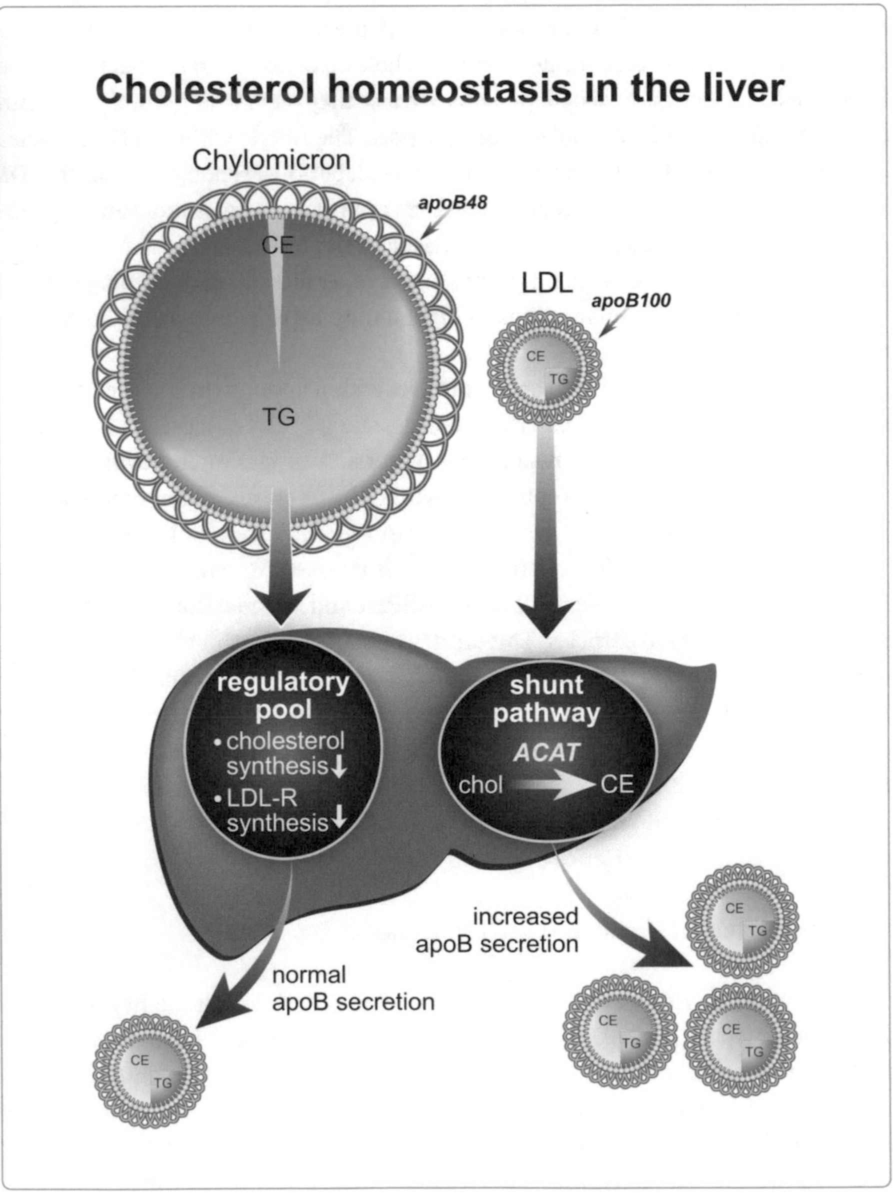

Cholesterol homeostasis in the liver

Finally, we suspect newly synthesized cholesterol tends to be either esterified and secreted or hydrolyzed by 7 alpha hydroxylase to bile acids. Thus in the fibroblast, cholesterol homeostasis is simple whereas in the hepatocyte it is complex with multiple discrete metabolic channels by which cholesterol passes into and through the cell and homeostasis is the sum of these.

1.4.4 Regulation of LDL Particle Number in Plasma

The concentration of LDL in plasma is determined by the rate at which LDL particles are produced and by the rate at which they are cleared. Each of these will now be briefly reviewed with the objective to demonstrate how changes in each affect the number of LDL particles in plasma.

1.4.4.1 Clearance

At steady state, by definition, the number of LDL particles produced per day must equal the number removed per day. The concentration of LDL particles – that is, the number per standard volume of plasma – will be determined both by the rate at which they are produced and by the efficiency of the processes that remove, or clear, them from plasma.[17,63] In brief, between 70 to 90% of LDL particles are removed by the liver per day by two different processes. The first involves uptake and removal of LDL particles by the LDL-receptor pathway. A specific region of the apoB molecule, which encircles the LDL particle, binds to the LDL receptor following which the complex is internalized within an endosome and delivered to a lysosome within the cell. Here, the apoB is hydrolyzed and the LDL receptor and the cholesterol within the particle released to the cytoplasm.

Regulation of the activity of the LDL-receptor pathway, as originally described by Brown and Goldstein,[63] is illustrated in Figure 1.24. In order to maintain cholesterol homeostasis, when the uptake of cholesterol within LDL particles into the cell increases (Figure 1.24 part A), a sequence of metabolic reactions, which are triggered by an increase in delivery of cholesterol to the endoplasmic reticulum, results in reduced synthesis of cholesterol and LDL receptors. In this model, increased intake of cholesterol therefore results in reduced production of cholesterol plus reduced capacity for subsequent intake of cholesterol. By contrast, reduced entry of cholesterol upregulates synthesis of cholesterol and LDL receptors (Figure 1.24 part B). However, as discussed above, whether this model applies within the hepatocyte is not clear since uptake of LDL does not result in the predicted downregulation of cholesterol synthesis.[62]

This simple teeter-totter homeostatic model was based on in vitro studies in human skin fibroblasts. Under these conditions, there is no option for cholesterol, which enters the cell to leave it. Whatever gets in must stay in. However, in contrast to the fibroblast in vitro, the hepatocyte in vivo has multiple options to export cholesterol including

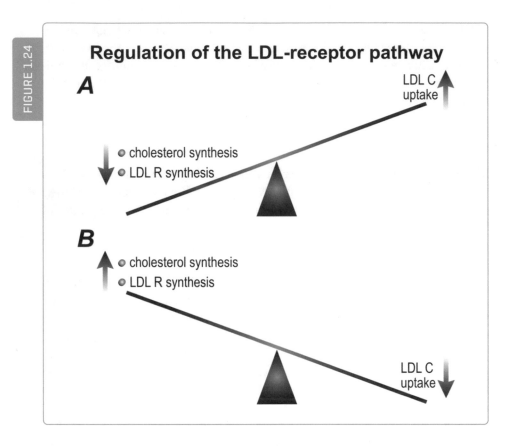

FIGURE 1.24

Regulation of the LDL-receptor pathway

A

LDL C uptake ↑

↓ ● cholesterol synthesis
● LDL R synthesis

B

↑ ● cholesterol synthesis
● LDL R synthesis

LDL C uptake ↓

secretion within apoB particles as well as transfer to nascent HDL particles. The hepatocyte is an infinitely more multifunctional cell than the fibroblast which is why the hepatocyte drives cholesterol balance physiologically and not the fibroblast. The simple teeter-totter homeostatic model does not seem to apply to the hepatocyte. Again, in particular, cholesterol and LDL-receptor synthesis seems to continue no matter how cholesterol is returned to the liver and this, as we will show below, changes the regulation of the concentration of LDL in plasma.

1.4.4.2 PCSK-9 Regulator of the LDL-Receptor

Unquestionably, the activity of the LDL-receptor pathway is a major determinant of the concentration of LDL particles in plasma and there is a direct relation between the number of LDL receptors on the cell surface and the activity of the pathway and therefore on the rate of removal of LDL particles and on LDL particle number in plasma. In a major recent discovery, it was appreciated that the protease, proprotein convertase subtilisin kexin type 9 (PCSK9), is an important independent determinant of the number of LDL receptors on the cell surface, and therefore the capacity to remove

LDL from plasma. PCSK9 is mainly synthesized in the liver, secreted into plasma and binds to some of the LDL receptors on the cell membrane surfaces. If a molecule of PCSK9 is attached to the LDL receptor, it will be hydrolyzed rather than recycled to the cell surface. Thus, PCSK9 is an important negative modulator of the number of LDL receptors on the cell surface of the hepatocytes. Inhibiting PCSK9 activity increases the number of LDL receptors on the cell surface and therefore increases the clearance of LDL particles from plasma. Multiple inhibitors of PCSK9 have been tested in initial trials in humans and all produce substantial decreases in plasma LDL C and apoB.

1.4.4.3 The LDL-Receptor Pathway and Non-Specific Pathways for Clearance of LDL from Plasma and their Effects on the Concentration of LDL in Plasma

To understand the regulation of the concentration of LDL in plasma, we must understand the performance characteristics of the LDL-receptor pathway in some detail.[17] The LDL-receptor pathway is a highly efficient uptake system but with a limited absolute capacity to transport LDL particles. Because LDL particles bind avidly to the LDL receptor, substantial numbers can be removed at relatively low concentrations. Unfortunately for us, because the LDL-receptor pathway is saturated at quite low levels of LDL in plasma, the absolute number of particles that can be removed by this route is limited.

If the production of LDL particles exceeds this limit, the so-called non-specific pathway must remove all the rest. These pathways remove a constant fraction of the LDL particles in plasma and this fraction is independent of the concentration of LDL particles in plasma. Thus, at low concentrations of LDL, the majority of clearance will be via the specific LDL-receptor pathway but a small minority will be cleared via the non-specific pathways. As concentrations of LDL increase, the non-specific pathways will remove more and more LDL particles.

To be in steady state, that is, for the concentration of LDL-C or apoB to remain the same day after day, the number of particles produced and the number removed must be the same. If, for any reason, the number of LDL receptors is reduced, but the production of LDL particles remains the same, the number of LDL particles removed must still equal the number of LDL particles that are being produced. Due to the reduction in the number of LDL receptors, the number that will be removed by the LDL-receptor pathway will be reduced. Therefore, the absolute number of LDL particles, which must be removed by non-specific pathways, will increase. Because this non-specific removal process is relatively inefficient, the number of particles in plasma will increase until the concentration of LDL particles is high enough that the non-specific pathways remove the necessary number.

This increase, however, will be substantial – much greater than one would intuitively imagine – because the non-specific pathways are not efficient. Similarly, but more commonly, if production of LDL particles increases, more must be cleared by non-specific pathways and, once again, there will be a disproportionately large increase in the number of LDL particles in plasma in order for this to occur. It is the disproportion in the change in concentration of LDL particles – relatively small changes in normal clearance will produce large changes in the number of LDL particles in plasma – that is key to understanding the concentration of LDL particles in plasma (Figure 1.25).

These principles we have just outlined are essential to understand and so we will present a simplified example. Let us say 1 LDL particle is produced per day and the fractional clearance rate of the LDL-receptor pathway is 50% or 0.500. This means that there must be 2 particles in the plasma pool for 1 to be cleared per day. Therefore, at a production and clearance rate of 1 LDL particle per day, the concentration of LDL particles in plasma will be 2 (Figure 1.25A). If the production rate increases to 2 particles per day but the LDL-receptor pathway can clear only 1 per day because its transport capacity is saturated, the extra particle will have to be cleared by the non-specific

FIGURE 1.25

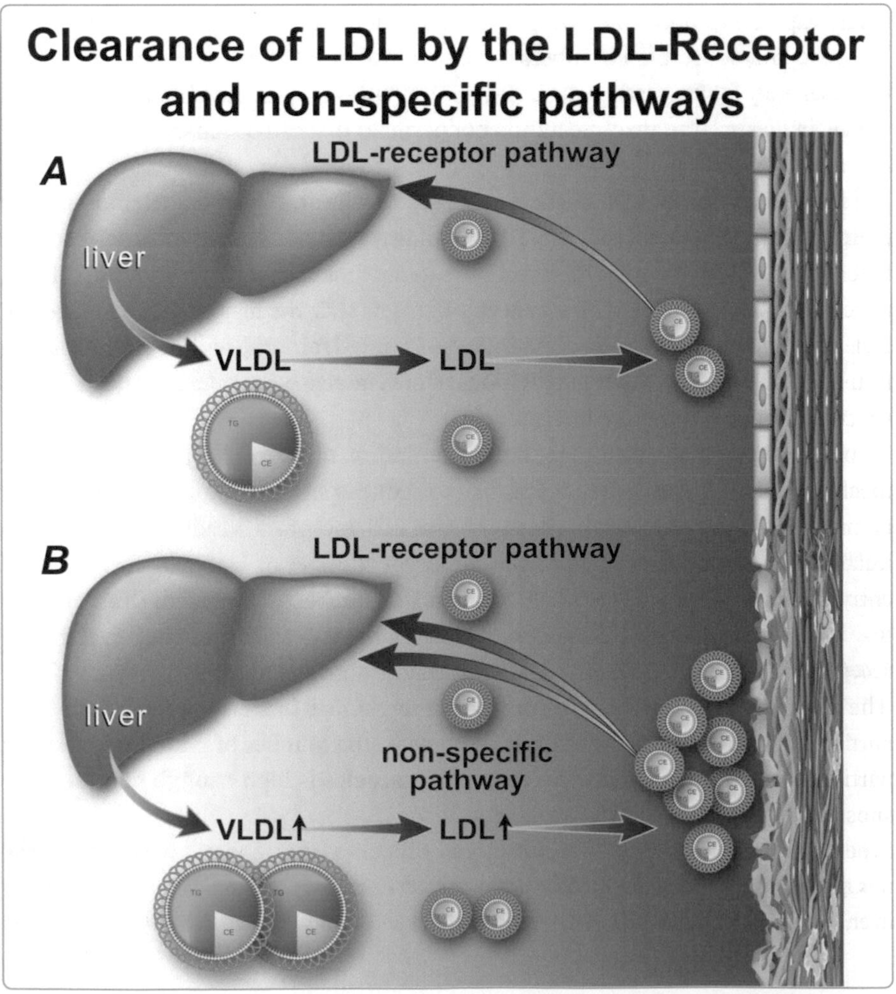

Clearance of LDL by the LDL-Receptor and non-specific pathways

A
LDL-receptor pathway
liver
VLDL → LDL

B
LDL-receptor pathway
liver
non-specific pathway
VLDL↑ → LDL↑

pathways. However, these pathways are less efficient than the LDL-receptor pathway. Their fractional clearance rate is only 20% or 0.200, which means there must be 5 LDL particles in the plasma compartment for one to be taken up by one of these mechanisms (Figure 1.25B).

Now let us do our sums. If the LDL-receptor pathway were not so limited in its absolute transport capacity and production increased to 2 particles per day, in order to clear 2 particles per day, the concentration would only increase to 4 particles per day. However, since this is not the case, the concentration will increase to 7 with 1 cleared by the LDL-receptor pathway and 1 by the non-specific pathways (Figure 1.25B). The point is that the increase in concentration is much greater than would be anticipated. A 100% increase in production resulted in a 350% increase in concentration. Similarly, a decrease in activity of the specific LDL-receptor pathway will also produce a sharp increase in the concentration of LDL in plasma.

Thus, either increased production or decreased clearance through the LDL-receptor pathway will sharply increase the concentration of LDL in plasma. The examples have been simplified to be comprehensible but the principles apply in real life. Importantly, when dealing with real life, it turns out that increasing production is an even more potent mechanism to increase concentration than reducing clearance and the most extreme elevations of LDL are due to a combination of increased production and decreased clearance through the LDL-receptor pathway. Nevertheless, whatever the mechanism that causes the number of LDL particles to increase, the artery 'sees' the concentration of LDL – the number of particles that are there. That is, the rate at which LDL particles enter and are deposited within the arterial wall is a direct function of the number of LDL particles in plasma. The transfer of apoB particles from the plasma space to the subintimal space of the artery is driven by the number of particles not by any specific metabolic process. That is why it is so important to understand the mechanisms that determine LDL particle number in plasma. To be sure, endothelial permeability does matter but changes in permeability are pathological not physiological. They also explain why apoB number is not the only determinant of apoB particle entry and atherogenic risk.

1.4.4.4 Secretion of VLDL/LDL

The rate at which LDL particles are produced is determined by the rate at which VLDL particles are secreted and by the rate at which VLDL particles are converted to LDL particles. The portion of VLDL particles that are converted to LDL particles varies substantially from very low in familial dysbetalipoproteinemia to very high in familial hypercholesterolemia. The determinants of this process are poorly understood, one of our most critical areas of ignorance. LDL particles can also be directly secreted by the liver, a phenomenon that is particularly prominent in familial hypercholesterolemia.[17]

The determinants of VLDL production are not well understood. More apoB molecules are synthesized than are incorporated into nascent VLDL particles and only a portion of nascent VLDL particles are secreted from the liver. Decreasing the proportion of apoB molecules that are hydrolyzed shortly after they are synthesized increases the proportion that are incorporated into nascent VLDL particles and therefore increases the rate at which VLDL particles are secreted by the liver (Figure 1.5). Similarly, increasing the proportion of nascent VLDL particles that are eventually secreted will positively affect the production rate of VLDL particles.

Almost all models of VLDL production favor a two-step process[12-15,71]: first, generation of a nascent lipid-poor apoB particle within the endoplasmic reticulum and then substantial expansion of the particle with addition of triglyceride within the Golgi. Microsomal triglyceride transport protein (MTP) plays an essential role in both these steps (Figure 1.5). Because triglycerides are the major lipid within VLDL particles, most presume VLDL secretion must be driven by the mass of triglycerides within the hepatocytes. And this may be so. Certainly, in general, although far from always, VLDL secretion is increased in the clinical disorders associated with increased hepatic triglyceride mass including abdominal obesity and type 2 diabetes mellitus.[13,72] Moreover, there is a large literature documenting a long list of factors for which there is in vitro or in vivo evidence that they affect triglyceride synthesis and secretion and/or apoB secretion. Amongst those that are most likely to be physiologically or pathologically significant are insulin, apoCIII, apoCII and perhaps apoAII. But these are only a few of molecules that have been shown to affect the balance between the proportion of newly synthesized apoB molecules that are incorporated into nascent particles versus the proportion hydrolyzed shortly after synthesis.

This detailed search is legitimate and interesting and is already obviously worthwhile, particularly in terms of apoCIII, but these are all factors that modify the rate at which the normal processes occur. We have chosen to focus elsewhere: namely, on the physiological raison d'être of the system, which is to transport lipids out of the hepatocyte. Specifically, because so much more cholesterol arrives in the liver than leaves in bile acids, we have chosen to focus on the potential role of cholesterol ester as a driver of apoB secretion. Addition of cholesterol ester in an MTP-driven process decreases the number of newly synthesized apoB molecules that are hydrolyzed before they are incorporated into nascent apoB particles.

VLDL secretion must be understood in terms of the number of particles that will be secreted and their composition. Much of the variance in composition is a function of the lipid loading of the particles. Increase the number of apoB particles that are secreted and the average mass of triglyceride per particle will decrease. Decrease this number and the average mass of triglyceride will increase. The critical consequence is downstream: the number of LDL particles that are produced. Familial combined hyperlipidemia is an example of VLDL particles of roughly normal composition being secreted at an increased rate whereas familial hypertriglyceridemia is an example of production of triglyceride-enriched particles at a normal rate.[73,74]

There is evidence that much of the cholesterol that drives apoB secretion is derived from cholesterol that has been taken up into the hepatocyte within LDL particles. Indeed, there appears to be a shunt pathway for cholesterol across the liver in which the cholesterol that enters the hepatocyte released from the lysosome is esterified by ACAT and secreted within VLDL apoB particles without ever coming into equilibrium with the regulatory pool of cholesterol within the endoplasmic reticulum (Figure 1.23).[62] This explains why hepatic cholesterol synthesis and synthesis of LDL receptors continue even though the liver receives far more cholesterol than it needs via uptake from LDL (Figure 1.25). This also explains why apoB secretion is increased in patients with heterozygous familial hypercholesterolemia and even more so in patients with homozygous familial hypercholesterolemia.[75] The increased apoB secretion with increased direct secretion of LDL as well as increased secretion of cholesterol-rich VLDL in turn, explains why the levels of LDL are so much higher than would be the case if absence of removal by the LDL-receptor pathway were the only metabolic abnormality.[65]

FA metabolism is usually considered separately from cholesterol metabolism but there is at least one important intersection: increased influx of FA to the liver increases not only triglyceride synthesis but also cholesterol ester synthesis (Figure 1.20 and Figure 1.26).[76] The consequences of this reaction are to increase the secretion rate of apoB particles and to increase hepatic synthesis of cholesterol. The synthesis of the molecule of cholesterol ester removes a molecule of cholesterol from the membrane of the endoplasmic reticulum and this molecule must be replaced; hence cholesterol synthesis must increase. Thus hepatic FA influx is an important determinant of plasma apoB and total body cholesterol mass (Figure 1.26).

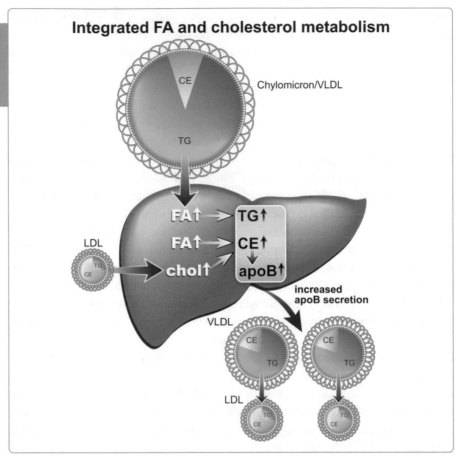

2. Diagnosis of the ApoB Dyslipo-
proteinemias: The ApoB Algorithm

- Excellence in clinical care begins with accurate diagnosis. Accurate diagnosis allows risk to be assessed most precisely and therapy to be chosen most appropriately.

- ApoB allows dyslipidemias to be redefined as dyslipoproteinemias. That is, the major lipids cholesterol and triglyceride – when integrated with apoB – allow apoB lipoprotein particle number and composition to be deduced. Clinical risk depends on which class of apoB lipoprotein particles is elevated.

- There are 6 different major apoB dyslipoproteinemias. With the exception of elevated Lp(a), all can be differentiated by the apoB algorithm based on total cholesterol, triglycerides and apoB and therefore each can be specifically identified and treated.

- Each of the apoB phenotypes can be a primary (i.e. genetic or familial) disorder or a secondary manifestation of another disorder.

- Using the apoB diagnostic algorithm not only leads to accurate diagnosis and more effective therapy in the individual, but any of the major familial dyslipoproteinemias can be recognized as well.

2.1 Introduction

Scientists are either lumpers or splitters. Lumpers group everything into the smallest number of categories possible. Splitters separate everything into as many categories as possible. In 1967, 5 articles in the NEJM, authored by Donald Fredrickson, Robert Levy and Robert Lees and entitled 'Fat transport in lipoproteins – an integrated approach to mechanisms and disorders' laid out a comprehensive and coherent classification of human dyslipidemia and established the clinical discipline of lipidology.[77-81] Based on LDL-C and triglycerides, these remarkable men, who wrote as well as they thought, identified distinct clinical presentations or phenotypes related to the different lipoprotein particles: chylomicrons, VLDL, IDL and LDL and remnant chylomicron and VLDL particles.

They based their classification on the lipoprotein particle phenotype. But they were limited by the technology of their times. They could not measure the number of the different lipoprotein particles. The apoB algorithm we present now is merely the physiological extension of the one they presented then with particle number added in.

Let us be clear. Fredrickson, Levy and Lees described phenotypes, which in certain instances linked closely to genotypes, but they never claimed that the phenotypes corresponded on each and every occasion, exactly and precisely, to individual, singularly distinct, definable genotypes. Nevertheless, it somehow became accepted wisdom that their classification was primarily genotypic rather than primarily phenotypic and, since this was clearly not the case, this was one major reason their scheme fell out of favor. Interest also evaporated because this approach could not explain why hypertriglyceridemia seemed to be highly atherogenic in some patients and in some families, whereas it was not in other patients and in other families. If the phenotype was the same, how could the outcome be so different?

Thus, dyslipidemia became simply hypertriglyceridemia, hypercholesterolemia or combined hypertriglyceridemia and hypercholesterolemia. Simplifying became accepted as the key to improving care and so the lumpers won and the work of Fredrickson, Levy and Lees, and the rationale on which it was based, has been largely lost. We disagree. The evidence indicates that clinical risk depends on which class of lipoprotein particles is elevated and evaluation of risk and decisions about therapy will be best when the diagnosis is most accurate.

Fredrickson, Levy and Lees had to base their diagnostic scheme on only two lipids: LDL-C and triglyceride. We now have the immeasurable advantage of having apoB, which accurately and easily measures the sum of VLDL and LDL particles and so we can come closer to separating the different patterns of lipoprotein particles: the apoB dyslipoproteinemic phenotypes. Accordingly, we will, in each case, define the phenotype based on the number and composition of the apoB lipoprotein particles that characterize it.

2.2 The ApoB Diagnostic Algorithm

The apoB dyslipoproteinemias are due to the elevation of one or more of the apoB containing lipoprotein particles: chylomicrons, VLDL particles, chylomicron and VLDL particles, remnant chylomicron and VLDL particles, LDL particles and Lp(a) particles. Recognizing elevated levels of Lp(a) requires a specific assay and therefore, elevated Lp(a) is the one atherogenic apoB dyslipoproteinemia that cannot be diagnosed by the apoB algorithm.[82] Other than Lp(a), however, the phenotypes for all the rest can be easily, accurately and instantly identified by the apoB algorithm from total cholesterol, triglycerides and plasma apoB, three tests that can be done in all routine biochemical laboratories.

Algorithms transform multiple, seemingly disconnected, pools of information into one final answer, providing – at least in principle – easy, accurate passage from complexity to simplicity. In this case, the apoB algorithm divides the apoB dyslipoproteinemias into a series of characteristic phenotypes, each produced by the excessive accumulation of one or more of the apoB lipoprotein particles. The diagnostic features of each phenotype are the consequence of the particle(s) involved, their number and their composition. Knowing which particles are present means knowing what clinical risks the patient faces and knowing which particles are present means knowing what treatment is best. Moreover, each phenotype may be due to primary abnormalities or secondary to other causes. Therefore knowing the phenotype provides insights into the causes of the phenotypes.

ApoB is an essential element of the algorithm. Using only cholesterol and triglycerides, patients with markedly elevated triglycerides due to chylomicrons cannot be distinguished reliably from those with markedly elevated triglycerides due to chylomicrons and VLDL particles. More important, they cannot be reliably distinguished from patients with markedly elevated numbers of chylomicron and VLDL remnants who are at markedly increased risk of vascular disease. Patients with moderately elevated triglycerides due to familial hypertriglyceridemia, who are not at substantially increased atherogenic risk, cannot be distinguished from patients with moderately elevated triglycerides due to familial combined hyperlipidemia, who are at tragically high risk.

All three – apoB, triglyceride and total cholesterol – can be measured in routine clinical chemistry laboratories using simple, inexpensive, automated procedures. Therefore, based on this diagnostic algorithm, the most advanced diagnoses can be made with the most basic measurements. Accordingly, this chapter will demonstrate how the 6 basic phenotypes can be differentiated based on total cholesterol, triglycerides and apoB and how this identifies the potential primary and secondary causes for each. Chapter 3 will present a more detailed characterization of the lipoprotein profile of each of the phenotypes as well as a description of their pathophysiological bases.

The ApoB algorithm

The architecture of the apoB algorithm is outlined in *the fly leaf of this book*. The origin and development of the algorithm has been published[82-85] and validated in different patient groups.[86-89] The apoB app, which can be downloaded for free from the internet, will automatically take you to the answer once you input total cholesterol, triglycerides and apoB. Total cholesterol and triglyceride can be entered either as mg/dl or mmol/l and apoB as either mg/dl or g/l.

• **HyperapoB: ApoB ≥ 1.2 g/l versus NormoapoB: ApoB < 1.2 g/l**

The first step divides the apoB lipoprotein particle disorders into those that typically present with HyperapoB, i.e., an apoB ≥ 1.2 g/l (120 mg/dl) versus those that typically present with NormoapoB, i.e., an apoB < 1.2 g/l.

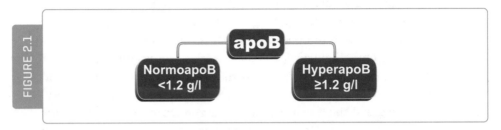

FIGURE 2.1

The level of 1.2 g/l was adopted as the level separating those with definitely elevated levels of apoB (i.e. ≥ 1.2 g/l) from those without definitely elevated levels because at that time it corresponded to the 75th percentile of apoB in the American population and also to the value that allowed the best diagnosis of patients with familial combined dyslipidemia. Subsequently, at least in the United States, the average levels of lipids and apoB have decreased and a level of apoB of 1.2 g/l now corresponds to the 90th percentile of the American population. However, we have maintained our original definitions and this will, of course, reduce the number classified as HyperapoB.

Nevertheless, the critical point, the point that must not be obscured by any classification, is that the actual level of risk attributable to apoB depends on the actual level of apoB. Risk increases exponentially as apoB increases. The risk attributable to an apoB of 1.15 g/l is not materially different from an apoB of 1.20 g/l.

• **NormoapoB: NormoTG < 1.5 mmol/l versus HyperTG ≥ 1.5 mmol/l**

Next, each of these categories – NormoapoB and HyperapoB – is subdivided into two groups on the basis of plasma triglyceride. A plasma triglyceride ≥ 1.5 mmol/l was chosen as the cut point because this is the level at which small cholesterol-depleted LDL particles become common. We will start with NormoapoB, which is divided into NormoTG NormoapoB and HyperTG NormoapoB.

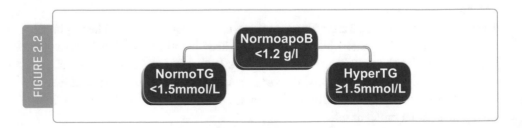

FIGURE 2.2

• NormoTG NormoapoB

NormoTG NormoapoB includes normal – those with normal lipids and normal apoB and two other phenotypes. First, an important variant of normal is an increased LDL-C ≥ 3.5 mmol/l (> 130 mg/dl) with a normal apoB (< 1.2 g/l), a phenotype that corresponds to a normal number of cholesterol-enriched particles. This phenotype is present in between 5-10% of the American population and is not associated with any increased cardiovascular risk over a 20-year follow-up period. Unless apoB is measured, these patients cannot be distinguished from those with elevated LDL-C and elevated apoB, who are at increased cardiovascular risk. Unless the correct diagnosis is made, unnecessary concern and treatment may well ensue. Second, an increased cholesterol, also without elevated apoB, can be due to increased LpX, the abnormal lipoprotein particles that are present in biliary cirrhosis and cholestasis and do not appear to convey any increased cardiovascular risk.

• HyperTG NormoapoB: TG/ApoB ≥ 10

The first step to separate the NormoapoB phenotypes with hypertriglyceridemia is to separate them based on TG/apoB ratio. Those with a TG/apoB ratio ≥ 10 (TG in mmol/l and apoB in g/l) are then subdivided into those with an apoB ≥ 0.75 g/l and those with an apoB < 0.75 g/l.

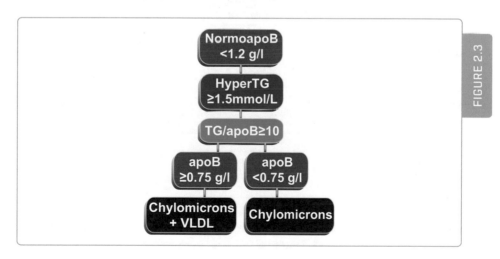

FIGURE 2.3

• HyperTG NormoapoB: TG/apoB ≥ 10 and apoB ≥ 0.75 g/l

Patients with a TG/apoB ≥10 and an apoB ≥ 0.75 g/l are characterized by an increased number of chylomicron and VLDL particles. Most commonly, this phenotype is present in those with a partial deficiency of lipoprotein lipase (LPL) plus a secondary factor such as diabetes mellitus, glucocorticoids, or estrogen therapy (further reading in Chapter 3 and 4). Typical values for this phenotype compared with normal are presented in Table

In table 2.1 to 2.6 average composition of all apoB and apoA lipoprotein particles in the six apoB dyslipoproteinemias are presented. A set of normal values has been compiled by the Lipid Clinic at Laval University and these are compared to those that are typical for the apoB dyslipoproteinemias.[75,88,204] The lipoproteins classes were separated by ultracentrifugation allowing composition to be determined for each.

Table 2.1 Average composition of all apoB and apoA1 lipoprotein particles in patients with hyperTG normoapoB due to the presence of VLDL and chylomicron particles.

	HyperTG normoapoB due to VLDL and chylomicrons (n = 101)	NormoTG NormoApoB (n = 440)
Age (yrs)	38.9±13.3	29.8±19.7
Gender (M/F)	81/20	240/200
Plasma Total Cholesterol mmol/l	8.23±4.17	4.99±0.84
Chylomicron-Cholesterol	4.75±3.39	—
VLDL-Cholesterol	1.66±1.20	0.34±0.16
LDL-Cholesterol	1.56±1.19	3.37±0.71
HDL-Cholesterol	0.61±0.18	1.28±0.36
Non-HDL Cholesterol	7.62±4.18	3.71±0.73
Plasma Triglycerides (TG) mmol/l	17.35±14.74	0.99±0.28
Chylomicron-TG	13.34±14.50	0.27
VLDL-TG	2.92±1.88	0.54±0.24
LDL-TG	0.50±0.23	0.23±0.07
HDL-TG	0.48±0.21	0.22±0.05
Plasma-apoB g/l	0.96±0.41	0.97±0.17
VLDL-apoB	0.26±0.17	0.097±0.04
LDL-apoB	0.70±0.32	0.87±0.16
HDL-apoAl g/l	1.04±0.27	1.25±0.23

2.1. Plasma total cholesterol is dramatically elevated as are plasma triglycerides. Plasma total cholesterol is elevated due to cholesterol in chylomicron and VLDL particles, whereas cholesterol in LDL and HDL particles is low. Plasma triglyceride levels are elevated due to the presence of an increased number of chylomicron and VLDL particles. Plasma apoB and LDL apoB are normal although VLDL apoB is twice normal. Given that cardiovascular risk is not substantially elevated in these patients, this argues against normal VLDL particles markedly increasing cardiovascular risk. In this and the other hypertriglyceridemic states LDL particles will be cholesterol depleted and triglyceride enriched whereas VLDL particles are cholesterol and triglyceride enriched.

• **HyperTG NormoapoB: TG/apoB ≥ 10 and apoB < 0.75 g/l**

Patients with a TG/apoB ≥ 10 and an apoB < 0.75 g/l are characterized by an increased number of chylomicron particles. The primary causes of this phenotype, which markedly increases the risk of pancreatitis, are complete deficiency of LPL or apoCII, the essential cofactor for lipoprotein lipase (LPL). Very unusual causes of this phenotype include systemic lupus erythematosus, due to antibodies which interfere with the action of LPL and defect in GPI-anchored HDL binding protein and apoAV deficiency (*further reading in Chapter 3 and 4*). Average values for affected patients compared with normal are given in *Table 2.2*. Whereas plasma triglyceride is profoundly elevated, indices of plasma cholesterol are not and apoB is frankly low. Plasma total cholesterol is the consequence of the cholesterol in an increased number of chylomicrons whereas the mass of cholesterol in LDL and HDL particles is profoundly low. Plasma triglycerides are elevated due to presence of the increased number of chylomicron particles, whereas the contribution of LDL and VLDL particles to plasma triglyceride levels is nil. Plasma apoB is low due to the very low number of LDL particles. These create the diagnostic features of the disorder.

Table 2.2 Average composition of all apoB and apoA1 lipoprotein particles in patients with hyperTG normoapoB due to the presence of chylomicron particles.

	HyperTG normoapoB due to chylomicrons (n–18)	NormoTG NormoApoB (n = 440)
Age (yrs)	33.5±14.3	29.8+19.7
Gender (M/F)	10/6	240/200
Plasma Total Cholesterol mmol/l	4.88±2.29	4.99±0.84
Chylomicron Cholesterol	3.36±2.90	—
VLDL-Cholesterol	0.23±0.13	0.34±0.16
LDL-Cholesterol	0.73±0.58	3.37±0.71
HDL-Cholesterol	0.41±0.17	1.28±0.36
Non-HDL Cholesterol	4.47±2.32	3.71±0.73
Plasma Triglycerides (TG) mmol/l	19.04±12.95	0.99±0.28
Chylomicron-TG	17.77±12.95	0.27
VLDL-TG	0.55±0.26	0.54±0.24
LDL-TG	0.35±0.12	0.23±0.07
HDL-TG	0.34±0.09	0.22±0.05
Plasma-apoB g/l	0.48±0.16	0.97±0.17
VLDL-apoB	0.07 ±0.04	0.097±0.04
LDL-apoB	0.42±0.16	0.87±0.16
HDL-apoAl g/l	0.80±0.15	1.25±0.23

• **HyperTG NormoapoB: TG/ApoB < 10**

Patients with hypertriglyceridemia and normal apoB but a TG/apoB ratio < 10 can be subdivided into those with a TC/apoB ≥ 6.2 and those with a TC/apoB < 6.2. Patients with a TG/apoB < 10 and TC/apoB ≥ 6.2 are characterized by an increased number of chylomicrons and VLDL remnants particles. Those with TG/apoB < 10 but TC/apoB < 6.2 have increased number of VLDL particles (*Figure 2.4*).

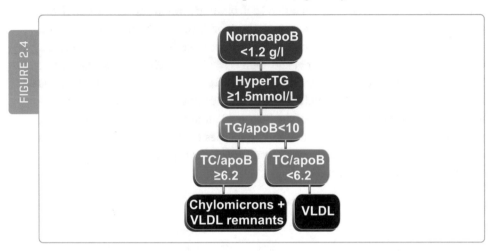

FIGURE 2.4

• **HyperTG NormoapoB: TG/ApoB < 10 and TC/ApoB ≥ 6.2**

The phenotype, remnant lipoprotein disorder, which is defined by increased numbers of chylomicron and VLDL remnants, is characterized by a TG/apoB < 10 and TC/apoB ≥ 6.2 (TC and TG in mmol/l and apoB in g/l). with a normal apoB. These abnormal remnant particles are not as triglyceride enriched as chylomicron particles but are cholesterol enriched compared with normal particles and are associated with a markedly increased risk of both coronary and peripheral vascular disease. Remnant lipoprotein disorder (or familial dysbetalipoproteinemia or type III dyslipoproteinemia) is a two hit disease, a genetic predisposition which may relate to an apoE2/E2 genotype (*see Chapter 3*) plus a secondary cause such as listed in the algorithm. Hepatic lipase deficiency also produces a genetic predisposition to this phenotype. This highly atherogenic lipoprotein phenotype, while unusual, is more common than previously thought and the apoB algorithm represents the only accurate clinically available tool for its diagnosis. If there were no other reason to measure apoB clinically, this would suffice.

Equally high levels of total cholesterol and triglyceride and a VLDL-C/triglyceride ratio > 0.69 mmol/l (> 0.3 mg/dl) are commonly suggested to indicate the presence of remnant lipoprotein disease. The typical lipoprotein profile is summarized in Table 2.3. Note that the average total cholesterol and triglyceride levels are not equal as is commonly thought. High plasma total cholesterol is due to very high amounts of

Table 2.3 Average composition of all apoB and apoA1 lipoprotein particles in patients with hyperTG normoapoB due to the presence of chylomicron and VLDL remnant particles.

	HyperTG normoapoB due to chylomicron and VLDL remnants (n=38)	NormoTG NormoApoB (n = 440)
Age (yrs)	44.2±11.0	29.8±19.7
Gender (M/F)	28/10	240/200
Plasma Total Cholesterol mmol/l	8.97±2.67	4.99±0.84
Chylomicron Cholesterol	—	—
VLDL-Cholesterol	5.59±2.94	0.34±0.16
LDL-Cholesterol	2.31±0.65	3.37±0.71
HDL-Cholesterol	0.91±0.24	1.28±0.36
Non-HDL-Cholesterol	8.06±2.76	3.71±0.73
Plasma Triglycerides (TG) mmol/l	6.13±3.78	0.99±0.28
Chylomicron TG	0.97	0.27
VLDL-TG	5.18+3.69	0.54±0.24
LDL-TG	0.42±0.11	0.23±0.07
HDL-TG	0.39±0.09	0.22±0.05
Plasma-apoB g/l	1.04±0.22	0.97±0.17
VLDL-apoB	0.44±0.18	0.097±0.04
LDL-apoB	0.60±0.15	0.87+0.16
HDL-apoAl g/l	1.26±0.24	1.25±0.23
VLDL-C/TG ratio mmol/l	0,9	0,34

cholesterol (high VLDL-C) in excessive numbers of VLDL particles (high VLDL-apoB), whereas cholesterol in LDL particles and the number of LDL particles (LDL-apoB) is normal or low. VLDL apoB, which in this case includes normal VLDL particles plus remnants of VLDL and chylomicron particles, is markedly elevated – fourfold higher than normal and the remnant particles are markedly enriched in cholesterol and triglyceride. Hopkins et al. have shown this disorder is much more common than generally appreciated.[25]

• HyperTG NormoapoB: TG/ApoB < 10 and TC/ApoB < 6.2
This phenotype is characterized by increased numbers of VLDL particles and a normal number of LDL particles. The atherogenic risk depends on the actual level of apoB and the presence or absence of other risk factors for cardiovascular disease, such as diabetes, which are listed in the algorithm. This disorder may be familial and the primary genetic abnormalities associated with this phenotype are partial LPL deficiency and apoAV deficiency.

Characteristic average values compared with normal are listed in *Table 2.4*. Plasma triglycerides are elevated due to increased number (high VLDL-apoB) of triglyceride-enriched VLDL particles (high VLDL-TG). Plasma total cholesterol is normal, but there is relatively more cholesterol in VLDL particles and relatively less in LDL and HDL particles. In the absence of high-risk features such as diabetes mellitus, cardiovascular risk is not markedly increased in these subjects, notwithstanding that VLDL apoB is twice normal.

Table 2.4 Average composition of all apoB and apoA1 lipoprotein particles in patients with hyperTG normoapoB due to the presence of VLDL particles.

	HyperTG normoapoB due to VLDL (n=433)	NormoTG NormoApoB (n = 440)
Age (yrs)	41.5±15.5	29.8±19.7
Gender (M/F)	310/123	240/200
Plasma Total Cholesterol mmol/l	5.05±0.95	4.99±0.84
Chylomicron.Cholesterol	—	—
VLDL-Cholesterol	1.50±1.15	0.34±0.16
LDL-Cholesterol	2.63±0.81	3.37±0.71
HDL-Cholesterol	0.91±0.28	1.28±0.36
Non-HDL-Cholesterol	4.14±0.91	3.71±0.73
Plasma triglycerides (TG) mmol/l	3.44±2.56	0.99±0.28
Chylomicron-TG	0.64±0.25	0.27
VLDL-TG	2.79±2.46	0.54±0.24
LDL-TG	0.32±0.09	0.23±0.07
HDL-TG	0.31±0.10	0.22±0.05
Plasma-apoB g/l	1.02±0.14	0.97±0.17
VLDL-apoB	0.21±0.10	0.097±0.04
LDL-apoB	0.81±0.17	0.87±0.16
HDL-apoAI g/l	1.15±0.23	1.25±0.23

• NormoTG HyperapoB: ApoB ≥ 1.2 g/l and TG < 1.5 mmol/l
This phenotype is characterized primarily by increased numbers of LDL particles. VLDL particle number may be increased but plasma triglycerides are not pointing to triglyceride-poor, cholesterol-rich VLDLIII particles. As indicated in the algorithm, there are multiple genetic causes, almost all of which are capable of producing marked increases in LDL particle number. Because clinical risk is determined by the phenotype not the genotype, genetic diagnosis is less important than recognition and therapy as well as screening of the rest of the family for others who might be affected. Second-

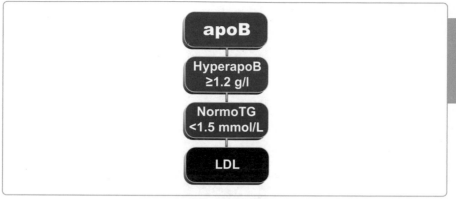

FIGURE 2.5

ary causes of this phenotype should always be considered including the nephrotic syndrome, hypothyroidism and perhaps anabolic steroids.

Typical values are listed in Table 2.5. The abnormalities are in LDL. The LDL particle number (LDL-apoB) is high as is LDL-C. The cholesterol content per LDL particle may be increased or average. Plasma triglycerides and HDL-C are, on average, normal.

Table 2.5 Average composition of all apoB and apoA1 lipoprotein particles in patients with normoTG hyperapoB due to the presence of LDL particles.

	NormoTG HyperApoB due to LDL (n=387)	NormoTG NormoApoB (n = 440)
Age (yrs)	33.2±19.6	29.8±19.7
Gender (M/F)	206/181	240/200
Plasma Total Cholesterol mmol/l	7.24±1.32	4.99±0.84
Chylomicron Cholesterol	0.4	—
VLDL-Cholesterol	0.36±0.16	0.34±0.16
LDL-Cholesterol	5.66±1.34	3.37±0.71
HDL-Cholesterol	1.22±0.34	1.28±0.36
Non-HDL Cholesterol	6.02±1.33	3.71±0.73
Plasma triglycerides (TG) mmol/l	1.04±0.27	0.99±0.28
Chylomicron-TG	—	0.27
VLDL-TG	0.51±0.23	0.54±0.24
LDL-TG	0.33±0.09	0.23±0.07
HDL-TG	0.20±0.04	0.22±0.05
Plasma-apoB g/l	1.47±0.26	0.97±0.17
VLDL-apoB	0.12±0.06	0.097±0.04
LDL-apoB	1.35±0.26	0.87±0.16
HDL-apoAI g/l	1.25±0.24	1.25±0.23

• HyperTG HyperapoB: ApoB ≥ 1.2 g/l and TG ≥ 1.5 mmol/l

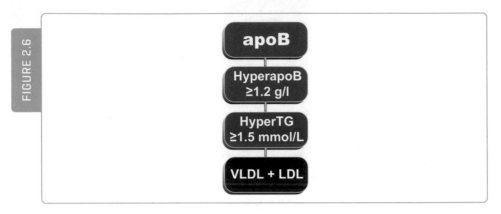

FIGURE 2.6

This phenotype is characterized by increased numbers of VLDL and LDL particles and is the commonest atherogenic phenotype associated with premature cardiovascular disease. Plasma triglycerides are elevated while total cholesterol and LDL-C may or not be increased. This phenotype is the hallmark of familial combined hyperlipidemia (FCH), the commonest proatherogenic familial dyslipoproteinemia. The phenotype is so common because so many of its provoking factors, as listed as secondary causes in the algorithm, are so common.

The average lipoprotein profile for affected patients is listed in Table 2.6. Plasma total cholesterol is elevated due, on the one hand, to an increased number of LDL particles, which increases LDL-C, and, on the other, to an increased number of VLDL particles that increases VLDL-C. Plasma triglyceride is elevated due to the presence of more VLDL particles (increase in VLDL apoB) resulting in high VLDL-TG.

2.3 Limitations of any Diagnostic Algorithm

Any diagnostic scheme comes with caveats. In the present instance, the most important are: first, while division into phenotypes enormously aids our appreciation of the metabolic mechanisms and relationships that determine plasma lipoprotein levels, any such division is artificial because the risk of vascular disease relates continuously to the number of atherogenic particles in plasma (apoB). There is no discrete point at which the level of plasma apoB is so high that it suddenly becomes 'abnormal' and none at which it poses zero risk. Moreover, in patients above as well as those below the boundary, risk varies: the higher the high apoB, the higher the risk; the lower the apoB, the lower the risk.

Table 2.6 Average composition of all apoB and apoA1 lipoprotein particles in patients with normoTG hyperapoB due to the presence of VLDL and LDL particles.

	HyperTG HyperApoB due to LDL and VLDL [n=763]	NormoTG NormoApoB [n = 440]
Age (yrs)	47.7±13.9	29.8±19.7
Gender (M/F)	512/251	240/200
Plasma Total cholesterol mmol/l	6.84±1.50	4.99±0.84
Chylomicron-Cholesterol	—	—
VLDL-Cholesterol	1.53+1.21	0.34±0.16
LDL-Cholesterol	4.36±1.42	3.37±0.71
HDL-Cholesterol	0.95±0.24	1.28±0.36
Non-HDL Cholesterol	5.89±1.48	3.71+0.73
Plasma triglycerides (TG) mmol/l	3.33±2.32	0.99±0.28
Chylomicron-TG	0.80±0.08	0.27
VLDL-TG	2.58±2.17	0.54±0.24
LDL-TG	0.47±0.19	0.23±0.07
HDL-TG	0.28±0.09	0.22±0.05
Plasma-apoB g/l	1.49±0.27	0.97±0.17
VLDL-apoB	0.24±0.12	0.097±0.04
LDL-apoB	1.25±0.28	0.07±0.16
HDL-apoAl g/l	1.18±0.21	1.25±0.23

Second, values are conventionally categorized as very high, high, high normal, normal or low based on where they fall within the overall distribution of values for a given population, these being > 90th percentile, the 75th-90th percentile, the 50th-75th percentile, the 10-50th percentile and < 10th percentile respectively. Since lipid levels including apoB levels differ in different regions of the world, these boundaries will differ also. But the relation to risk will remain: societies with higher average apoB levels will have higher incidence rates of vascular disease than societies with lower average apoB levels.

Third, total personal risk relates to the total profile of the major risk factors in the individual, not simply to the level of the proatherogenic and antiatherogenic lipoproteins. Nevertheless, so long as these reservations are kept in mind, as we will demonstrate, the apoB algorithm can be of considerable clinical value.

3. The Primary ApoB Dyslipoproteinemias

In this chapter, we will review the pathophysiology, clinical features, diagnostic criteria and treatment of the primary apoB dyslipoproteinemias. Importantly, all these apoB dyslipoproteinemic phenotypes can be simply and accurately distinguished by the apoB algorithm.

Overview of the primary apoB dyslipoproteinemias

1 HyperTG NormoapoB due to chylomicrons
- Complete LPL deficiency
- Primary apoCII deficiency
- Defect in GPI-anchored HDL binding protein
- apoAV deficiency

2 HyperTG NormoapoB due to chylomicrons and VLDL
- Partial LPL deficiency with secondary factors
- ApoAV deficiency

3 HyperTG NormoapoB due to chylomicrons and VLDL remnants
- Familial dysbetalipoproteinemia or remnant lipoprotein disorder
- Hepatic lipase deficiency
- Primary cause associated with a secondary factor

4 HyperTG NormoapoB due to VLDL particles or TG-enriched VLDL particles
- Familial hypertriglyceridemia
- Partial LPL deficiency
- ApoAV deficiency

5 HyperTG HyperpaoB due to VLDL and LDL particles
- Familial combined hyperlipidemia
- Sitosterolemia

6 NormoTG HyperapoB due to LDL particles
- Familial hypercholesterolemia
- Familial defective ApoB
- PCSK9 gain of function
- Autosomal recessive hypercholesterolemia
- Polygenic hypercholesterolemia
- CYP7A1 deficiency
- Hypoalphalipoproteinemia
- Cholesterol ester storage disease

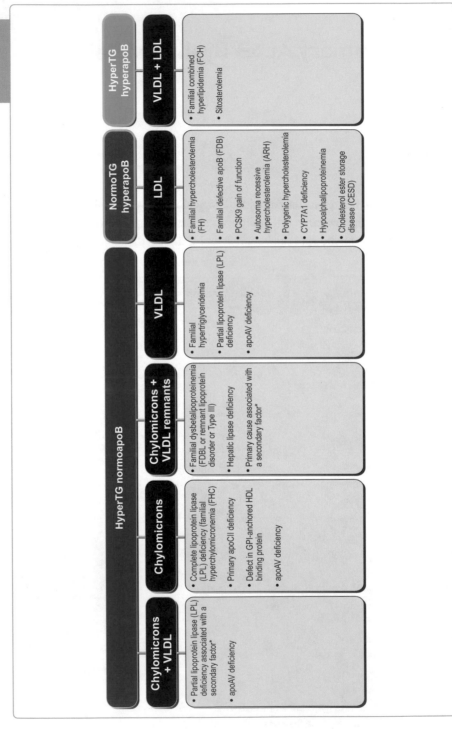

FIGURE 3.1

HyperTG normoapoB

Chylomicrons + VLDL
- Partial lipoprotein lipase (LPL) deficiency associated with a secondary factor[a]
- apoAV deficiency

Chylomicrons
- Complete lipoprotein lipase (LPL) deficiency (familial hyperchylomicronemia (FHC)
- Primary apoCII deficiency
- Defect in GPI-anchored HDL binding protein
- apoAV deficiency

Chylomicrons + VLDL remnants
- Familial dysbetalipoproteinemia (FDBL or remnant lipoprotein disorder or Type III)
- Hepatic lipase deficiency
- Primary cause associated with a secondary factor[a]

VLDL
- Familial hypertriglyceridemia
- Partial lipoprotein lipase (LPL) deficiency
- apoAV deficiency

NormoTG hyperapoB

LDL
- Familial hypercholesterolemia (FH)
- Familial defective apoB (FDB)
- PCSK9 gain of function
- Autosoma recessive hypercholesterolemia (ARH)
- Polygenic hypercholesterolemia
- CYP7A1 deficiency
- Hypoalphalipoproteinemia
- Cholesterol ester storage disease (CESD)

HyperTG hyperapoB

VLDL + LDL
- Familial combined hyperlipidemia (FCH)
- Sitosterolemia

3.1 HyperTG NormoapoB

This can be due to (*Figure 3.1*):
1) Increased chylomicron particles
2) Increased chylomicron particles and increased VLDL particles
3) Increased chylomicron and VLDL remnants particles
4) Increased VLDL particles

3.1.1 HyperTG NormoapoB due to Increased Chylomicron Particles

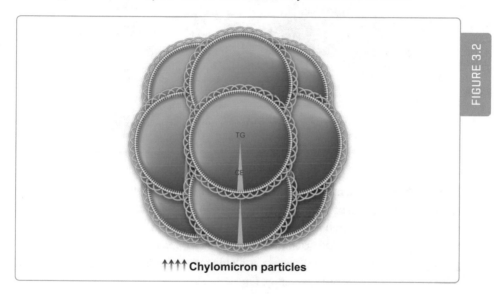

FIGURE 3.2

↑↑↑↑ **Chylomicron particles**

Diagnosis
Hyperchylomicronemia is present in patients with marked hypertriglyceridemia (triglycerides > 6 mmol/l) in combination with an apoB < 0.75 g/l and a TG/apoB ≥ 10.[90-94] The combination of very high triglycerides and low apoB is the key to diagnosis.

Pathophysiology
Chylomicrons are the largest, most triglyceride-rich apoB particles and are synthesized and secreted by the intestine. The triglyceride within chylomicrons is normally rapidly hydrolyzed by lipoprotein lipase (LPL) in adipose tissue and skeletal muscle and the remnant particle that is produced, which contains some of the original triglyceride and all of the original cholesterol, is then rapidly removed by the liver (*Figure 3.3 and see Figure 1.2*). Because each chylomicron particle contains so much triglyceride – a chylomicron particle can reach 1200 nm or 8000 angstroms in size (*see Table 1.1*) – it requires only a relatively small number of chylomicron particles to produce very elevated triglyceride levels.

FIGURE 3.3

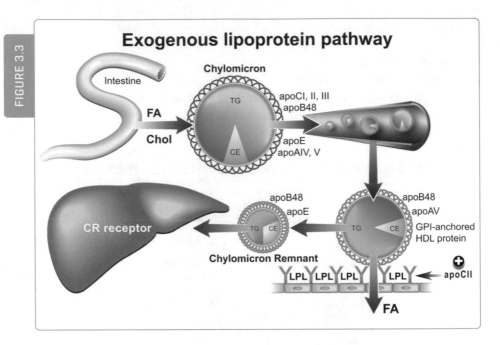

In hyperchylomicronemia, the total apoB is strikingly low. The low total apoB is predominantly the effect of a low LDL apoB. The LDL particles appear to be enriched in triglyceride and depleted in cholesterol (*see Table 2.2*); HDL-C is low: all findings, which might be anticipated given the high plasma triglyceride levels and therefore the greatly increased mass of triglyceride available for cholesterol ester transfer protein (CETP)-mediated core lipid exchange (*Figure 1.12*).

Causes

The principal genetic cause of marked hyperchylomicronemia is failure to synthesize active LPL (*Figure 3.4*).[90,92] Most cases are compound heterozygotes due to mutations in exons 5 and 6 of the LPL gene and involve either the catalytic or the heparin-binding domain. A mutation in apoCII, an essential co-factor for LPL activity, is a less common but also well-established cause of this syndrome. A few cases have been related to a defect in glycophosphatidylinositol (GPI-) anchored HDL binding protein, a protein, whose function is to bind LPL to the endothelium[95] and there is considerable interest in the critical role that apoAV may play in triglyceride clearance from plasma (*Figure 3.5*).[96]

Clinical Diagnosis

Hyperchylomicronemia is rare: approximately 1 per 1 million in the population. Chylomicrons are too large to penetrate the vascular wall with any facility and so vascular

FIGURE 3.4

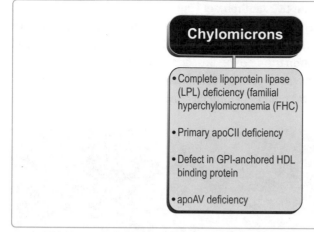

Chylomicrons

- Complete lipoprotein lipase (LPL) deficiency (familial hyperchylomicronemia (FHC)

- Primary apoCII deficiency

- Defect in GPI-anchored HDL binding protein

- apoAV deficiency

FIGURE 3.5

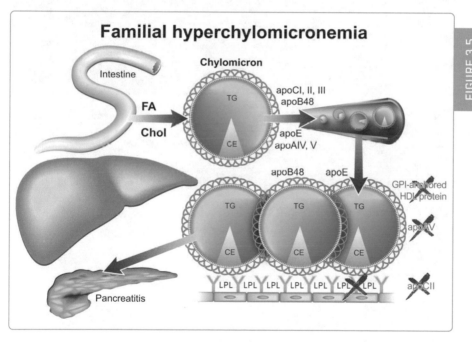

Familial hyperchylomicronemia

Intestine

Chylomicron

FA

Chol

TG

CE

apoCI, II, III
apoB48

apoE
apoAIV, V

apoB48   apoE

TG   TG   TG

CE   CE   CE

GPI-anchored HDL protein

apoAV

LPL LPL LPL LPL LPL LPL LPL

apoCII

Pancreatitis

disease is not a problem. Rather, pancreatitis is the clinical risk from severe hyperchylomicronemia with microvascular obstruction due to the chylomicron particles a popular hypothesis. The risk becomes substantial when plasma triglyceride levels are more than 10 mmol/l. However, some patients will not develop pancreatitis even with triglyceride levels as high as 100 mmol/l whereas others suffer acute pancreatitis at triglyceride levels of 5 mmol/l.

A major clinical feature is eruptive xanthomata (Figure 3.6), small, yellowish-white papules that often appear in clusters, on the back, buttocks, and extensor surfaces of the arms and legs. Lipemia retinalis is another major clinical feature – the retinal blood vessels on fundoscopic examination are opalescent as shown in Figure 3.7 which disappears after treatment of the hypertriglyceredimia (Figure 3.8). Finally, hepato-splenomegaly due to the uptake of circulating chylomicrons by reticuloendothelial

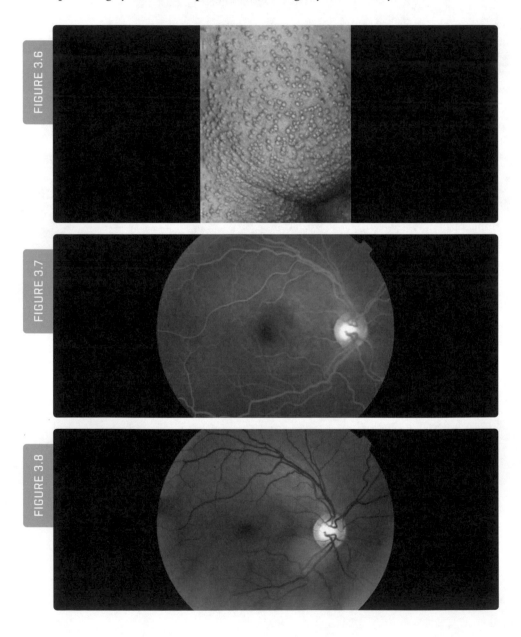

FIGURE 3.6

FIGURE 3.7

FIGURE 3.8

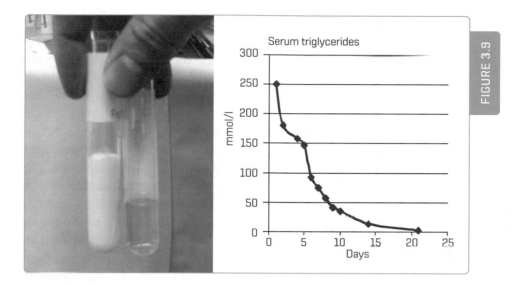

FIGURE 3.9

cells in the liver and spleen can be found on physical examination. A blood sample may appear pale and the serum milky (Figure 3.9). Pseudohyponatremia may be present but this is less likely given newer laboratory methods. Occasionally plasma must be diluted in order to recognize the true extent of the elevated triglycerides.

Since triglyceride levels tend to decrease substantially in the first 48 hours after the onset of pancreatitis, delay in presentation may obscure diagnosis of this as the cause of the acute pancreatitis. Large increases in serum amylase may not be present and an elevated pancreatic lipase may, in fact, be a more reliable indicator of the problem.[92] Imaging with MRI or CT that demonstrates intrapancreatic or peripancreatic edema is the most reliable tool to diagnose the pancreatitis. The initial attack of acute pancreatitis may result in pseudocysts, which increase the potential for further clinical episodes.

Treatment

Fasting for at least 24 hours is the first priority in treatment for patients with acute pancreatitis due to hyperchylomicronemia. When there is no dietary intake of cholesterol and triglycerides, no chylomicrons will be formed, and triglycerides will fall to within the normal range within days (Figure 3.9) Intravenous fluids are administered as necessary and plasmapheresis can be considered if available and if the patient is critically ill. An insulin drip may be effective to improve activity of LPL even when blood glucose is not elevated. For patients not admitted to hospital, the major therapeutic intervention in familial chylomicronemia syndromes is dietary fat restriction (to as little as 15 g/day to limit the formation of chylomicrons) with fat-soluble vitamin supplementation.

Long-term management of these patients involves lifestyle changes (avoidance of alcohol, weight reduction and low-fat diet). The value of medium-chain triglycerides needs to be better defined as clinical reports of their efficacy differ.[97] Medications are often considered in patients with fasting plasma triglyceride levels > 10 mmol/l with a target of triglycerides < 5 mmol/l. Unfortunately, medications such as fibrates generally do little. Management of patients with familial chylomicronemia syndrome is particularly challenging during pregnancy and may require plasmapheresis to remove the circulating chylomicrons (*See also Table 4.5, Chapter 4*). The EVOLVE (Epanova for Lowering Very High Triglycerides) study reported success with the free fatty acid (FA) form of omega-e FA in severe hypertriglyceridemia.[98] Of considerable interest is a report documenting marked reductions in plasma triglycerides in 3 patients who were either homozygotes or compound heterozygotes for LPL deficiency with infusion of an inhibitor of apoCIII messenger RNA.[99] Given that apoCIII is thought to inhibit LPL activity, which is genetically absent in most of these patients, these positive results are welcome, but surprising, and indicate how much remains to be learned about triglyceride clearance from plasma. Work is underway to develop a gene therapy approach[100] and at least acute therapy with a microsomal triglyceride transport inhibitor such as lomitapide might be considered.[101]

3.1.2 HyperTG NormoapoB due to Elevated Chylomicrons and VLDL Particles

Diagnosis
These patients have marked or severe hypertriglyceridemia (triglycerides > 6 or 10 mmol/l) due to increased numbers of chylomicrons and VLDL particles (*Figure 3.10*). The triglyceride-rich particles account for a triglyceride/apoB ratio ≥ 10 and the syndrome is distinguished from pure hyperchylomicronemia by an apoB > 0.75 g/l. Most of these patients have a normal apoB but the occasional patient has an elevated value due to an associated increase in LDL particle number (*see Table 2.1*).

Pathophysiology
As well as chylomicrons, LPL hydrolyzes triglycerides in VLDL particles, which is the first step in their conversion to LDL particles. An increase in VLDL production is thought to saturate triglyceride clearance. If this occurs, even modest increases in production will produce profound increases in plasma triglycerides.

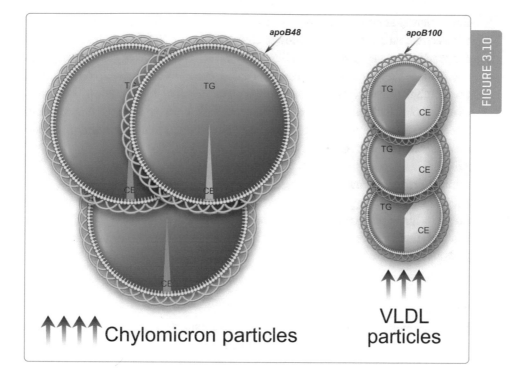

FIGURE 3.10

apoB48

apoB100

TG

TG

TG

CE

CE

CE

TG

CE

TG

CE

CE

↑↑↑↑ Chylomicron particles

↑↑↑ VLDL particles

Causes

There are no known primary causes for this disorder but it can be associated with a partial LPL deficiency or an abnormality in apoAV, an apolipoprotein, which appears to be involved in the association of LPL with triglyceride-rich particles (Figure 3.11).

However, when partial LPL or apoAV deficiency is associated with a secondary factor, such as abdominal obesity, type 2 diabetes mellitus (DM2), alcohol abuse, or medica-

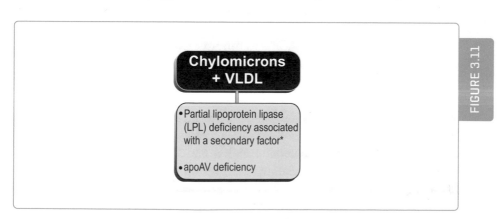

FIGURE 3.11

Chylomicrons + VLDL

• Partial lipoprotein lipase (LPL) deficiency associated with a secondary factor*

• apoAV deficiency

tions such as steroids or estrogens or isotretinoin (Accutane), then severe hyper-triglyceridemia due to accumulation of chylomicron and VLDL particles may result. Pregnancy[92] can also provoke the clinical expression of this phenotype. Beta-blockers and thiazide therapy have also been implicated. If beta-blocker therapy is required, the metabolic side effect profile of agents such as carvedilol is preferable to those such as metoprolol. In these patients, triglyceride clearance is already severely compromised. Therefore, relatively modest increases in VLDL production can produce profound increases in plasma triglyceride levels.

Clinical Presentations

Patients with severe hypertriglyceridemia due to chylomicrons and VLDL particles may present with eruptive xanthomata and plasma may appear milky (*see Figures 3.6, 3.7, 3.8 and 3.9*). If chylomicron and VLDL particle numbers are increased sufficiently, pancreatitis may occur. Plasma apoB is only occasionally elevated above the 75th percentile (i.e. > 1.2 g/l).

Treatment

In patients with severe hypertriglyceridemia who are at risk of pancreatitis, dietary total fat intake should be reduced acutely. Secondary causes should be identified and, if present, treated. Treatment with fibrates or omega-3 FA may be helpful in these patients, particularly when plasma triglycerides have fallen due to restriction of fat intake if partial LPL activity is present. Nicotinic acid is also an option. If the patient is diabetic, an insulin drip may be helpful. Whether LDL-lowering therapy with statins is indicated depends on the level of apoB and the clinical circumstances. Patients with increased cardiovascular risk because of the presence of DM2 or a history of cardiovascular disease (CVD) will require LDL-lowering therapy to reduce apoB levels to at least < 0.75 g/l and, if appropriate to < 0.65 g/l (*see Chapter 6*). The same range of options is available to treat the severe hypertriglyceridemia in these patients as in those with hyperchylomicronemia (*see 3.1.1 and Table 4.3 Chapter 4*).

3.1.3 HyperTG NormoapoB due to Remnant Lipoprotein Disorder

Diagnosis

In patients with combined hypercholesterolemia and hypertriglyceridemia and normal apoB, one should always consider whether remnant lipoprotein disorder is present. The diagnostic criteria in the apoB algorithm are: apoB < 1.20 g/l, TG ≥ 1.5 mmol/l, triglyceride/apoB < 10, total cholesterol/apoB ≥ 6.2. Characteristic for remnant lipoprotein disorder is the accumulation of chylomicron and VLDL remnant particles (*Figure 3.12*).

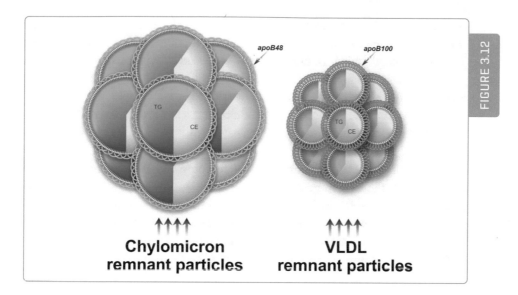

FIGURE 3.12

**Chylomicron
remnant particles**

**VLDL
remnant particles**

Pathophysiology

As outlined in Chapter 1, the triglyceride-rich lipoproteins, chylomicrons and VLDL are metabolized in two steps: first, the bulk of the triglycerides are removed in peripheral tissues and second, and almost immediately thereafter, the products of the first step, known as remnant lipoprotein particles, are removed by the liver (*See Figure 1.14, 1.5 and 1.6*). In *Figure 3.13* the normal endogenous lipoprotein pathway is presented.

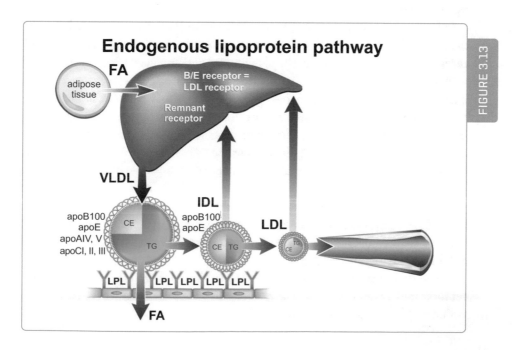

FIGURE 3.13

Because these normal remnant particles are removed so rapidly, they are present in only small numbers in plasma – one-tenth or less the number of VLDL particles in the peak postprandial period. Drastic failure of the second step is the hallmark of this phenotype and leads to the accumulation of modified highly atherogenic remnant particles within plasma – 20 to 40 fold above normal.

The normal removal process for chylomicron remnants is complex and has many interconnected parts, including multiple enzymes – hepatic lipase and lipoprotein lipase – multiple proteins with receptor-like functions, such as the LDL-receptor related protein (LRP) and the putative VLDL receptor, and other potentially critical components of the membrane, such as heparin sulfate proteoglycans and apoE. The processes by which VLDL particles are either removed from plasma or converted to LDL particles are even more complex and less well understood. In both instances, it appears that the particles must associate with the external membrane of the hepatocytes and apoE has been thought to be one of the important elements involved in this process.

Causes

ApoE2/E2 Mutation: Frederickson, Levy and Lees labelled this disorder type III hyperlipo-proteinemia;[102] others have designated it familial dysbetalipoproteinemia (FDBL).[25,26] We prefer the term remnant lipoprotein disorder. Whatever the label, this disorder injures and kills those that it affects and does so rapidly and with no remorse. That is the dark side of this diagnosis. The other side, the bright side, the side of hope, is that this phenotype is eminently treatable, which means that making the diagnosis in time can be life-saving.

Indeed, a characteristic genotype – apoE2/E2 – has been thought to be a hallmark of remnant lipoprotein disorder (*Figure 3.14*). ApoE2 has a lower affinity for the hepatic receptor, which removes normal chylomicron and VLDL remnants, than the two other alleles of apoE: apoE3 and apoE4. Other rare mutations in apoE were associated with a dominant form of FDBL where the hyperlipidemia is fully manifest in the heterozygous state. More recently, however, it has become clear that an apoE2/E2 genotype is present only in about 30% of patients with phenotypic positive remnant lipoprotein disorder indicating the pathophysiology must be reconsidered.[25] Actually, it has been known for some time that the apoE2/E2 phenotype alone (approximately 1% of the population) is not sufficient to produce the full clinical syndrome which is present in only 1/50 or less of E2/E2 individuals. An additional provoking factor must be present to produce the full clinical syndrome. The most common of these are a high-fat diet, diabetes mellitus, obesity, hypothyroidism, renal disease, estrogen deficiency, alcohol use, or certain drugs (*Figure 3.14*).

Whatever the actual reason for their impaired clearance, if VLDL particles are not removed rapidly from the plasma, they necessarily circulate for much longer periods within it and consequently, by virtue of CETP-mediated core lipid exchange with HDL

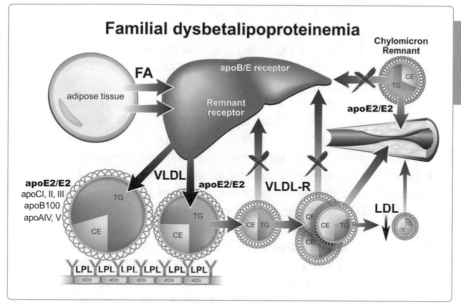

FIGURE 3.14

Familial dysbetalipoproteinemia

and LDL particles, become cholesterol-enriched abnormal remnant lipoprotein particles (see Figure 1.12). Because each abnormal remnant particle contains substantial amounts of cholesterol and triglyceride, marked hypercholesterolemia and hypertriglyceridemia are the lipid hallmarks of this phenotype. Because only a small fraction of VLDL particles is metabolized to produce LDL particles, the number of LDL particles – LDL apoB – is strikingly reduced. The total apoB is characteristically normal due to a reciprocal striking increase in the number of remnant chylomicron and VLDL particles.[25,88] Whereas normally, VLDL particles make up only 10% of total apoB particles and LDL particles make up 90%, in remnant lipoprotein disorder, LDL makes up approximately 60% and the remnants 30 to 40%, so 20-40 fold more than normal. It is the staggering increase in remnant particle number that accounts for the profound increase in cardiovascular risk (see Table 2.3).

Clinical Diagnosis

Unfortunately, from the conventional standard panel of lipid tests, the diagnosis can be suspected but not made. These patients have combined hyperlipidemia with classically marked elevations of both triglycerides and cholesterol. Rough equality (if expressed in mg/dl), if present, is suggestive but not much more. However, more recent data demonstrate triglyceride and cholesterol levels may be only moderately elevated.[25] Moreover, the traditional advanced approaches to diagnosis of this disorder, lipoprotein electrophoresis (broad beta band) or ultracentrifugation (ratio of VLDL-C to total plasma triglyceride > 0.30 mg/dl or > 0.69 mmol/l), are not generally available even in specialty laboratories. ApoE genotyping does identify E2/E2 homozygotes for apoE2. However, absence of the apoE2/2 genotype does not rule out the diagnosis whereas presence of the apoE2/E2 genotype does not mean a particular dyslipidemia is actually remnant disorder. Indeed only a minority of cases of documented remnant disorder are E2/E2 genotype.

Fortunately, diagnosis is now simple using the apoB algorithm and can be made in any laboratory that measures total cholesterol, triglycerides and apoB. Indeed, if there were only one reason to measure apoB, making the diagnosis of this malignant metabolic disorder a practical objective for every clinical laboratory would suffice. Given the high vascular risk of remnant disorder, diagnosis is an indication for therapy.

Peripheral vascular disease is a major feature in these patients as well as coronary artery disease (CAD). Why disease in these vessels is so prominent in this disorder but not in familial hypercholesterolemia (FH) is, to the best of our knowledge, an important question that remains unasked and therefore unanswered. Moreover, we know that remnant lipoprotein disorder is uncommon in women before menopause but we do not know why it is so much more common after.[25] Two distinctive types of xanthomas, tubero-eruptive and palmar, are seen in FDBL patients: tubero-eruptive xanthomas (Figure 3.15 (before) and 3.16 (after treatment)), which begin as clusters of small papules on the elbows, knees, or buttocks and can enlarge to the size of small grapes and palmar xanthomas, which are orange-yellow discolorations of the creases in the palms and wrists (Figure 3.17).

Treatment

Remnant lipoprotein disorder should be treated aggressively. As a first step, any condition that is known to precipitate the expression of remnant lipoprotein disorder, such as obesity, DM2, significant alcohol intake and hypothyroidism should be identified

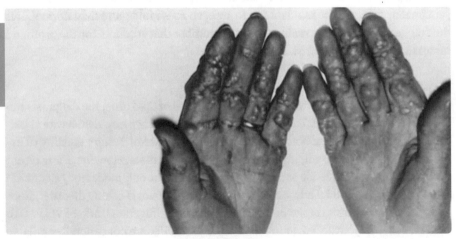

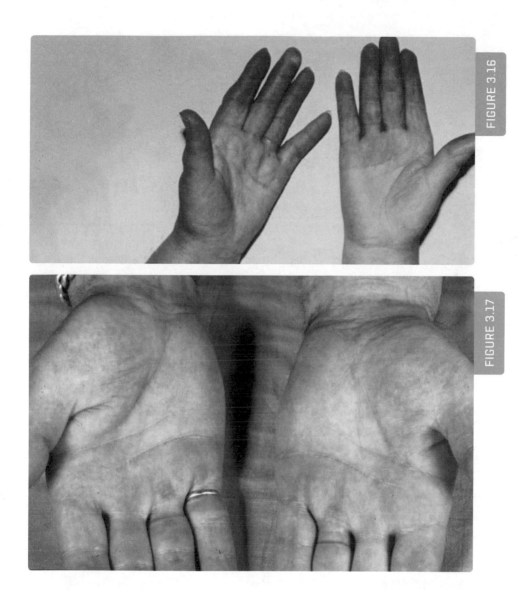

FIGURE 3.16

FIGURE 3.17

and treated. Patients with remnant disorder typically respond favorably to weight reduction and to low-cholesterol, low-fat diets. Alcohol intake should be curtailed and estrogen treatment stopped. Pharmacological treatment is aimed at decreasing the number of atherogenic remnant particles. In this instance, risk would be severely underestimated if total plasma apoB were relied on. Treatment should aim at normal levels of cholesterol and triglyceride and apoB levels < 0.65 g/l. Patients with remnant lipoprotein disorder may respond well to fibrates as well as statins or even niacin. Occasionally, combination drug therapy is required (*see also Table 4.4, Chapter 4*).

FIGURE 3.18

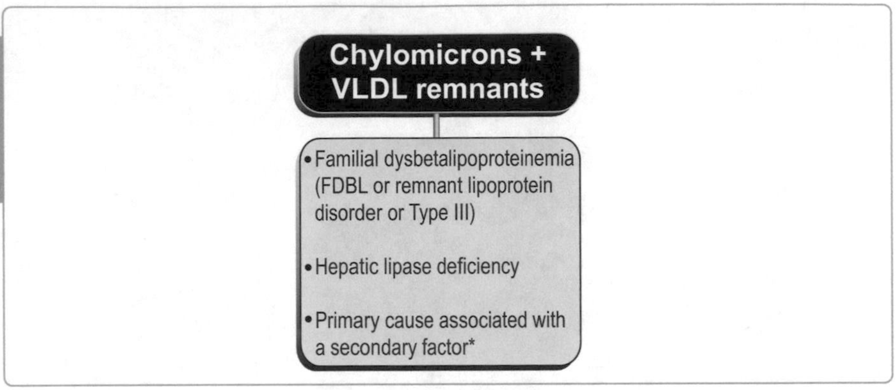

Hepatic Lipase Deficiency: Hepatic lipase deficiency is a rare autosomal recessive disorder, which may produce the remnant lipoprotein disorder phenotype.[103]

Hepatic lipase is involved in the conversion of VLDL to LDL particles; therefore, hepatic lipase deficiency results in increased numbers of chylomicron and VLDL remnants. Phenotypic diagnosis is made by application of the apoB algorithm and, if resources are available, confirmed by measuring hepatic lipase activity in post-heparin plasma. Diet, fibrates or statins remain the appropriate therapies. Finally chylomicrons and VLDL remnants may be due to a primary cause associated with a secondary factor (Figure 3.18).

3.1.4 HyperTG NormoapoB due to Increased VLDL

Diagnosis
An increased size and/or increased number of VLDL particles with a normal number of LDL particles produces mildly or moderately elevated triglyceride levels, a normal plasma apoB and VLDL particles that are not profoundly triglyceride or cholesterol enriched (Figure 3.19). Diagnosis using the apoB algorithm includes triglyceride ≥ 1.5 mmol/l; triglyceride/apoB < 10; total cholesterol/apoB < 6.2; apoB < 1.20 g/l.

Pathophysiology
Hypertriglyceridemia in these patients is due either to triglyceride-enriched VLDL particles or to an increased number of VLDL particles of normal composition or both. (see Figure 3.19) Because the rate at which VLDL particles are secreted is normal, the rate at which LDL particles are formed is normal: therefore total plasma apoB is not elevated (< 1.20 g/l). Hypertriglyceridemia may result either if the particles that are secreted by the liver are enriched in triglycerides or, alternatively, if the production of VLDL particles is normal, but the clearance rate is reduced resulting in the accumulation of VLDL particles and therefore elevation of plasma triglycerides. Thus, HyperTG NormoapoB is characterized by an increased number of triglyceride-enriched VLDL particles with a normal apoB (see Table 2.4).

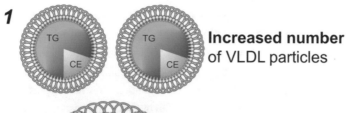

FIGURE 3.19

Hypertriglyceridemia due to increased number or size of VLDL particles

1 — **Increased number** of VLDL particles

TG CE
TG CE

2 — **Increased size** of VLDL particles

TG CE

Causes (Figure 3.20)

– *Familial Hypertriglyceridemia* (FHTG) is a relatively common (∼1 in 500) autosomal dominant disorder of unknown etiology although a disorder in bile acid metabolism has been suggested.[104] Increase in breakdown of newly synthesized cholesterol by 7-alpha hydroxylase might reduce the mass of cholesterol esters at the smooth endoplasmic reticulum, decreasing the rate at which apoB particles are preserved after they are formed, resulting in the secretion of fewer but more triglyceride-enriched VLDL particles.

– *Partial LPL Deficiency.* Partial LPL deficiency may be present in heterozygous carriers of LPL mutations and in carriers of common gene variants in the LPL gene.[105]

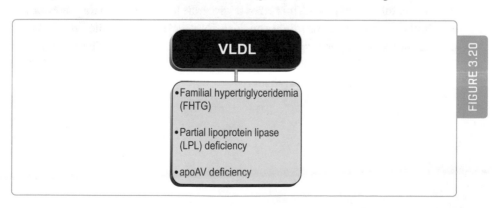

FIGURE 3.20

VLDL

- Familial hypertriglyceridemia (FHTG)
- Partial lipoprotein lipase (LPL) deficiency
- apoAV deficiency

– *ApoAV Deficiency:* ApoAV is an apolipoprotein, which appears to be required for the association of VLDL and chylomicrons with LPL or may work as an activator of LPL.[106]

Such patients present with a normal or a modestly increased number of VLDL particles with a normal number of LDL particles. Since LDL particles are so much more numerous than VLDL particles, apoB is normal and cardiovascular risk is not substantially increased. However, if associated with a secondary factor such as abdominal obesity, DM2, alcohol or medication such as steroids or estrogens, then severe hypertriglyceridemia due to accumulation of chylomicron and VLDL particles may result (*see Chapter 4*).

Clinical Diagnosis
Hypertriglyceridemia due to VLDL is a biochemical diagnosis with no specific clinical manifestations. As plasma triglycerides usually do not exceed 6 mmol/l, the risk of pancreatitis is low. Because total apoB is not markedly elevated i.e. < 1.2 g/l, cardiovascular risk due to the apoB lipoproteins is not markedly increased in such patients. The identification of other first-degree relatives with hypertriglyceridemia is useful in making the diagnosis FHTG.

Treatment
As an isolated finding, increased VLDL particles do not require pharmacological therapy. Moreover because the number of atherogenic particles is not increased (apoB < 1.2 g/l), the atherogenic risk of this dyslipoproteinemia attributable to apoB is not marked. However, this dyslipoproteinemia is commonly found in patients with associated high-risk abnormalities. If the overall risk of vascular disease were increased sufficiently, as it would be in patients with DM2, then pharmacological therapy would definitely be indicated. If so, statins should be the primary therapy to reduce apoB to the appropriate target level, < 0.75 g/l in high-risk and < 0.65 g/l in very high-risk patients. Multiple drugs are unlikely to be required. Ezetimibe can be used in patients who do not tolerate statins. As increased triglyceride levels are the main presentation of this phenotype, clinicians might consider fibrates. However, while fibrates lower triglyceride levels, they only modestly lower the number of atherogenic apoB particles and there is insufficient randomized clinical trial evidence to justify their use in this phenotype (*see also Table 4.2, Chapter 4*).

3.2 HyperTG HyperapoB due to Increased VLDL and LDL Particles

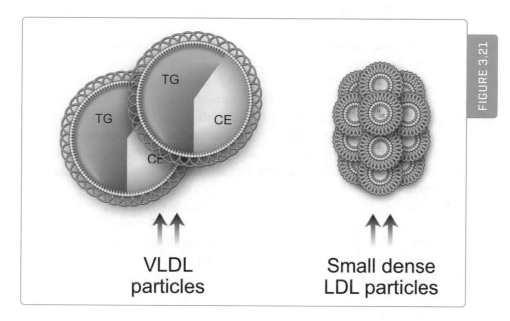

FIGURE 3.21

VLDL particles

Small dense LDL particles

Diagnosis

These patients have a triglyceride ≥ 1.5 mmol/l and therefore they are hypertriglyceridemic. They may or may not be hypercholesterolemic, but they all have an apoB ≥ 1.20 g/l and therefore they all have an elevated LDL particle number. The main causes are indicated in Figure 3.22.

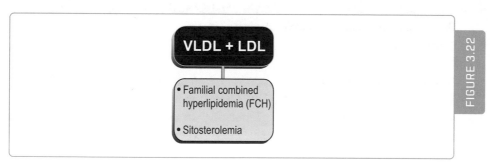

FIGURE 3.22

3.2.1 Familial Combined Hyperlipidemia (FCH)

Four decades ago, FCH was recognized by three different investigative teams and defined as an inherited lipid disorder characterized by the presence of multiple lipoprotein phenotypes – hypertriglyceridemia, hypercholesterolemia or both – within a family. FCH was found to be strongly associated with premature CVD and is, by far, the commonest atherogenic familial hyperlipidemia yet described, affecting 1% to 5.7% of the adult population and up to 20% of patients with premature myocardial infarction.[107-109]

However, it soon became clear the lipid phenotype could vary over time in affected individuals including, at least in some, periods of apparent normalcy of cholesterol and triglyceride. Despite its prevalence and despite the potent linkage between FCH and accelerated CVD, the diagnosis of FCH is almost never made in clinical care. How could it be that this disease, the commonest familial disorder associated with premature coronary artery disease (premature CAD), has become, for all practical purposes, a disease that has been lost, a disease now known only to those who continue to study it and not to most of those who suffer from it or to those who should be able to diagnose and treat it?

The first reason is that the concept was inherently contradictory: how could one disease cause so many different phenotypes and how could they come and go? Second, as originally defined, the diagnosis is much too challenging in routine clinical practice. Different lipid phenotypes must be present in a family, which means that the family must be large enough and the members old enough, since elevated lipids are not common in subjects with FCH until the third decade or later. Third, in contrast to FH, no simple, straightforward, elegant molecular causal explanation for FCH has been identified.

Fourth, patients with hypertriglyceridemia due to FCH were at increased cardiovascular risk whereas those with hypertriglyceridemia due to FH were not.[110,111] But why was this so? Or, starting the other way around, which patients with hypertriglyceridemia had FCH and were therefore at high cardiovascular risk and which had familial hypertriglyceridemia and were at low cardiovascular risk? All these shortcomings have caused FCH to fade from clinical consciousness but not from clinical expression and clinical consequence.

New Diagnostic Criteria for FCH: ApoB ≥ 1.2 g/l and TG ≥ 1.5 mmol/l

In 2002, a working group redefined FCH based on pathophysiology and used apoB as well as lipids to characterize the phenotype.[112] In a series of studies, De Graaf and colleagues showed that the FCH phenotype could be defined as a plasma triglyceride >1.5 mmol/l and a plasma apoB > 1.20 g/l.[113-115]

As would be anticipated, increased numbers of small dense cholesterol-depleted LDL particles were a prominent feature of the dyslipoproteinemia in these patients as was a lower HDL-C (*see Figure 3.23*). Thus, HyperTG HyperapoB is the diagnostic phenotype of FCH, all of which corresponded to the phenotype of HyperTG HyperapoB. By contrast, HyperTG NormoapoB is the phenotype that corresponds to familial hypertriglyceridemia.[116]

Metabolic Pathways Involved in FCH

With the new diagnostic criteria, FCH became a single phenotype with a clear, coherent and consistent pathophysiology.[117] We will now discuss briefly the causes involved in the different metabolic pathways (Figure 3.23 and Figure 3.24).

– Hepatic Metabolism in FCH

Elevated hepatic secretion of VLDL apoB particles is the hallmark functional abnormality in FCH.[74] Increased secretion of VLDL apoB particles produces an elevated VLDL particle number, exceeding the normal capacity to clear VLDL triglycerides. Hence elevated triglycerides were a primary feature. The second cardinal feature was an elevated plasma apoB. The increased secretion of VLDL particles led to an increased production of LDL particles as VLDL particles were converted into LDL particles, hence the elevated apoB. An increased number of triglyceride-rich VLDL particles and perhaps an increased activity of cholesterol ester transfer protein results in most of the LDL particles being smaller and cholesterol depleted.

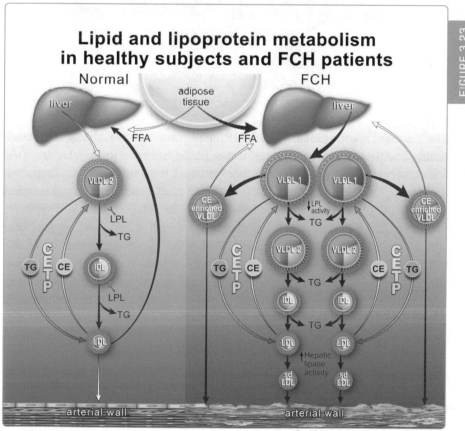

Lipid and lipoprotein metabolism in healthy subjects and FCH patients

FIGURE 3.23

FIGURE 3.24

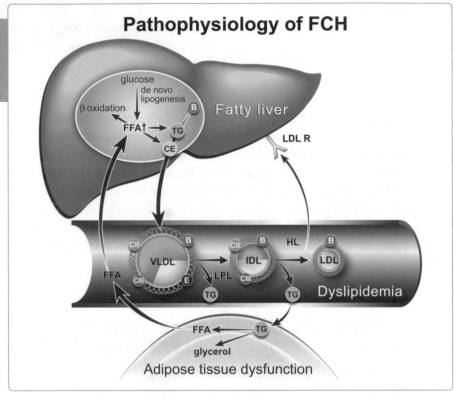

Pathophysiology of FCH

The increased hepatic production of VLDL apoB particles is most likely, most commonly, a consequence of an increased flux of FA the liver and a principal cause of the increased hepatic FA flux is abdominal obesity, which is often associated with glucose intolerance, insulin resistance and DM2 (*see Figure 3.24*). However, FCH can manifest in childhood, generally as an elevated apoB without frank hyperlipidemia.[118] Typically, FCH is not fully expressed until the third or fourth decade of life, which suggests that age-related environmental factors, such as the typical age-related expansion of adipose tissue mass, contribute to the full phenotypic expression of FCH in individuals who already have an underlying primary abnormality, perhaps in hepatic sterol metabolism.[119,120] This stepwise natural history may well be abbreviated by the increasing prevalence of obesity in the young.

– Dysfunctional Adipose Tissue and Abnormal Free FA Metabolism
Because adipose tissue dysfunction is key to the pathophysiology of FCH, understanding in more detail the regulation of the flux of FA into and out of adipocytes is essential to understand the increased hepatic apoB secretion in FCH (*Figure 3.23*) as also outlined in *Chapter 1.3* and shown in *Figure 1.14 and 1.15*.

Abnormal free FA metabolism in FCH has been demonstrated in vivo with reduced FA trapping by adipocytes producing increased FA flux to the liver.[52,121] Methodologically elegant and physiologically powerful studies of triglyceride storage and release from adipocytes by Arner and his colleagues clearly document significant functional abnormalities consistent with reduced FA trapping and increased FA release by adipocytes and high FA flux to the liver in subjects with FCH and elevated apoB.[122-124] These functional abnormalities include reduced activity of the ASP pathway,[51] insulin resistant adipose tissue metabolism,[125] resistance to the lipolytic effects of catecholamines due to a defect in HSL or to insulin resistance or to the effects of a number of hormones and adipocytokines, such as leptin, TNF alpha, adiponectin, which themselves have been suggested to be causes or consequences of insulin resistance/visceral obesity.[126,127]

The role of these adipocytokines in the pathogenesis of FCH needs further investigation.

Combining whole genome expression profiling data in adipose tissue, followed by pathway analyses, has identified other differential and potentially causal pathways in FCH including the upregulated complement pathway[128] and overrepresentation of cell cycle genes, which might functionally contribute to dysfunctional adipogenesis in FCH.[129]

Genetic Determinants of FCH

Much effort has been expended to identify the genetic origins of FCH. The original model of FCH as an autosomal dominant disorder is not sustainable and FCH has evolved into a complex multifactorial disorder, the outcome of the interaction of multiple major and modifying genes. In our review on the genetics of FCH, we provide a comprehensive overview of the genes that have been implicated in FCH and its associated traits, including an indication of the level of corroborating evidence such as from linkage studies.[130] Currently up to 35 genes have been described, a number of which have been implicated in the various aberrant metabolic pathways in FCH (see Figure 3.24). However, there are a substantial number of genes reported to be associated with FCH or FCH-related traits, for which the exact roles remain to be determined. Accordingly, a major challenge in FCH research is to connect these genes to metabolic effector pathways and, vice versa, to identify new genes for pathways known to be aberrant in FCH.

One of the most-replicated genes in FCH is the transcription factor upstream stimulatory factor 1 (USF1). USF1 has numerous target genes, including those related to lipid and glucose metabolism. Unfortunately, the exact molecular mechanisms by which genetic variance in USF1 contributes to the etiology and phenotype of FCH has remained elusive. One piece of this puzzle that was recently resolved is that USF1 variants may affect hepatic triglyceride metabolism by modulating the microsomal triglycerides transfer protein expression.[131] Using whole exome sequencing, Rosenthal et al. identified the mitochondrial membrane transport protein SLC25A40 as a potentially causal factor for hypertriglyceridemia in a large FCH pedigree, thus revealing a novel metabolic pathway and a potential novel treatment target for hypertriglyceridemia.[132]

We recently identified PCSK9 as a heritable trait in FCH[133] although the gene(s) responsible for elevated PCSK9 levels have not yet been identified, nor did the Genome-Wide Association Study reveal a significant association in the general population.[134]

However both PCSK9 expression and cholesterol synthesis are affected by SREBP2, and FCH patients manifest elevated markers of cholesterol synthesis,[135-137] which are correlated with PCSK9 levels.[138] These findings point towards SREBP2 as an attractive upstream candidate for the expression of PCSK9 in FCH.

Multiple innovative genetic strategies to identify potential causal pathways in FCH are becoming available, including whole genome expression profiling in specific target organs, followed by pathway analyses. Using this approach, we recently demonstrated upregulation of the complement pathway in subcutaneous adipocytes of FCH patients.[128] However, meaningful integration of large, multi-dimensional datasets derived from genomics, metabolomics, clinical and imaging datasets is currently one of the major challenges in the life sciences. Overcoming this bottleneck is essential if we are ever to understand the complex biological systems that underlie this complex disease.

Treatment of FCH

Individuals with FCH should be treated aggressively due to the significantly increased risk of premature CAD. Decreased dietary intake of saturated fat and simple carbohydrates, aerobic exercise, and weight loss can all have beneficial effects on the lipid profile. Weight reduction can produce substantial improvements in the lipoprotein profile and should be strongly recommended and supported. Patients with diabetes should be aggressively treated to maintain good glucose control. Most patients with FCH require lipid-lowering drug therapy to reduce atherogenic apoB lipoprotein levels to the recommended range and therefore to reduce the high risk of CVD. Statins are effective but some patients will need a second drug (a cholesterol absorption inhibitor most often) for optimal control of apoB levels. Pharmacological therapy with fibrates added to statins has been suggested to reduce triglycerides and increase HDL-C in very high-risk patients. However, clinical trial results have not supported this combination, albeit the subjects were not selected for this phenotype. Several intervention trials, such as the ACCORD study, have suggested that the combination of fibrates and statins may be beneficial in patients with elevated plasma triglycerides (> 2.3 mmol/l) and low HDL-C levels.[139] However, these are post facto analyses. Niacin has long been regarded as an alternative lipid-lowering drug to combine with statins. However, the recently reported AIM-HIGH and HPS-2 THRIVE studies have demonstrated that extended-release niacin is not of additional benefit to prevent cardiovascular complications when combined to statin therapy.[140] Finally, the hitherto described heritable and increased levels of circulating PCSK9 in FCH make FCH patients good candidates to receive PCSK9 antagonizing therapy.[133,138] Phase 2 studies have shown that mono-clonal antibodies directed against circulating PCSK9 are well tolerated and result in an impressive LDL cholesterol-lowering effect, even on top of statin therapy (*see also Table 4.1, Chapter 4*).[141]

3.2.2 Sitosterolemia

Pathophysiology
In normal individuals, < 5% of dietary plant sterols (i.e. sitosterol and campesterol) are absorbed by the proximal small intestine and delivered to the liver. Sitosterolemia is a rare autosomal recessive disease in which the intestinal absorption of plant sterols is increased and biliary excretion of the sterols is reduced, resulting in increased plasma and tissue levels of sitosterol and other plant sterols.[142] Sitosterolemia is caused by mutations in one of two members of the ATP-binding cassette (ABC) transporter family, ABCG5 and ABCG8.[143] The trafficking of cholesterol is also impaired in sitosterolemia as the total amount of bile acid produced from cholesterol is reduced because secretion of cholesterol into the bile is retarded. Due to the reduced secretion of bile acids, cholesterol synthesis is reduced. Therefore, bile acid resins and, at the extreme, ileal bypass surgery are effective therapies whereas statins are not.

Clinical Diagnosis
Sitosterolemia is confirmed by demonstrating an increase in the plasma level of sitosterol using gas chromatography. Cholesterol levels in patients with sitosterolemia range from normal to high. In homozygotes, apoB tends to be disproportionately high compared with cholesterol. In heterozygotes apoB values are not increased. Patients develop tendon xanthomas (*Figure 3.25 (before)* and *Figure 3.26 (after treatment)*) as well as premature atherosclerosis and can be mistaken for FH patients. Episodes of hemolysis, presumably secondary to the incorporation of plant sterols into the red blood cell membrane, are a distinctive clinical feature of this disease.

Treatment
The dyslipoproteinemia in subjects with sitosterolemia is unusually responsive to reductions in dietary cholesterol content. Sitosterolemia should be suspected in patients in whom the plasma cholesterol level falls more than 40% on a low-cholesterol diet. The dyslipoproteinemia does not respond to statins. However, bile acid sequestrants and cholesterol-absorption inhibitors, such as ezetimibe and a diet low in phytosterols, are the best options.

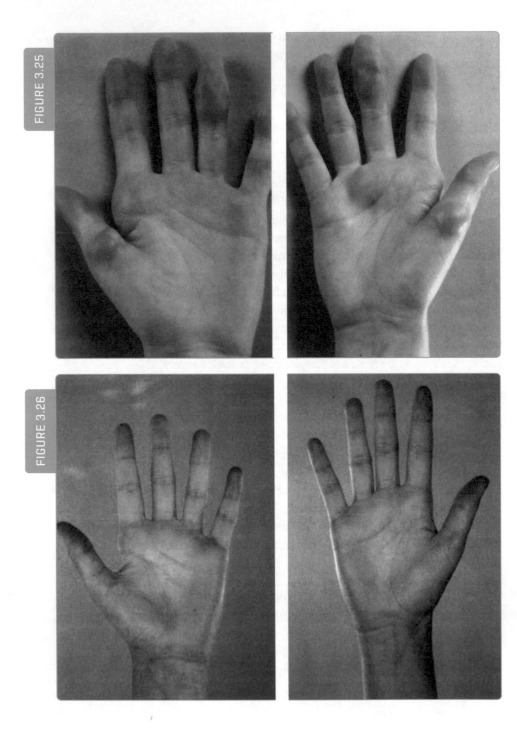

3.3 NormoTG HyperapoB due to Increased LDL Particles

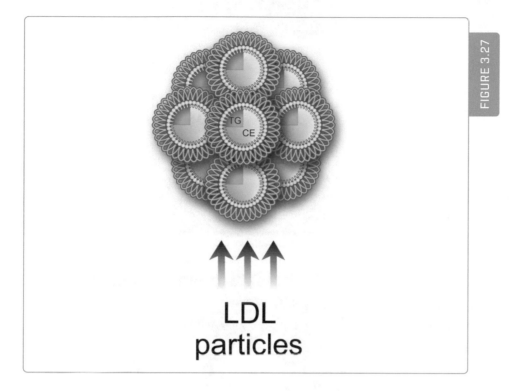

FIGURE 3.27

Diagnosis

This phenotype is characterized by an increase in LDL particle number and therefore in atherogenic risk. Characteristically, but not universally, the LDL particles tend to be cholesterol enriched or of normal composition. Thus, both LDL-C and apoB are elevated. Triglycerides by definition are normal and this reflects the fact that impaired clearance is, characteristically, the prime physiological abnormality but this is generally coupled with increased hepatic apoB secretion, either as VLDLIII or directly as LDL. The disorders in this category vary in their clinical severity (Figure 3.28).

3.3.1 Severe Hypercholesterolemic Phenotype

The severe hypercholesterolemic phenotype is at the extreme end of the spectrum.[64] These patients have massively elevated levels of LDL and present with the clinical syndrome of FH. There are multiple genetic causes of the clinical phenotype of FH (Figure 3.29). Most represent monogenic disorders, most often due to functional mutations in the LDL receptor, less frequently due to mutations in apoB or PCSK9. The clinical phenotype is similar for all.[144-146] Diagnosis of the clinical phenotype calls for family

FIGURE 3.28

LDL

- Familial hypercholesterolemia (FH)
- Familial defective apoB (FDB)
- PCSK9 gain of function
- Autosoma recessive hypercholesterolemia (ARH)
- Polygenic hypercholesterolemia
- CYP7A1 deficiency
- Hypoalphalipoproteinemia
- Cholesterol ester storage disease (CESD)

FIGURE 3.29

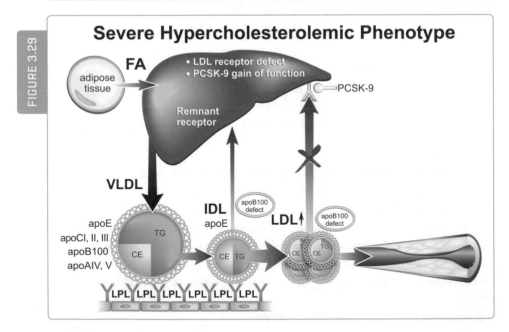

Severe Hypercholesterolemic Phenotype

screening. The controversy is whether this should be accompanied by genetic screening. However, it is now clear that the same clinical phenotype can result from a polygenetic mechanism of inheritance, which can also be expressed in other family members. This makes the value of genetic cascade screening questionable as there is no clear evidence so far as the lipoprotein status is concerned that risk in these patients is related to anything other than the level of LDL.

3.3.1.1 Heterozygous FH (HeFH)

Heterozygous Familial Hypercholesterolemia (HeFH) occurs in 1 in 500 persons worldwide, making it one of the commonest clinically significant monogenic disorders. Patients with HeFH have high LDL from birth. In several countries, cascade family screening programmes are being organized to identify children and young adults before irreversible arterial damage has occurred. When this is not available, the disease is often not detected until adulthood with routine cholesterol screening or the appearance of tendon xanthomas (*Figure 3.30 and 3.31*) or the development of symptomatic coronary atherosclerotic disease.

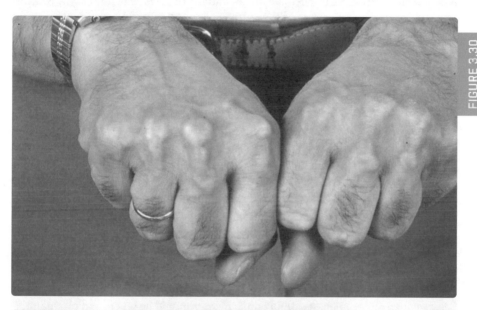

FIGURE 3.30

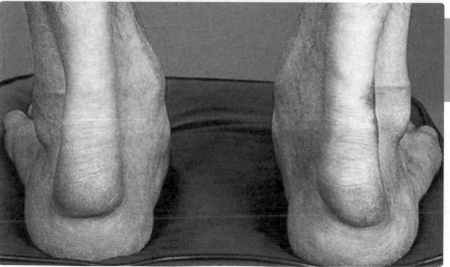

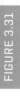

FIGURE 3.31

Clinical Diagnosis

HeFH is characterized by a markedly elevated LDL particle number as reflected by high apoB (1.50-2.00 g/l) and high LDL-C (usually 5.2-10.0 mmol/) and normal levels of triglyceride. Levels of Lp(a) are typically higher than normal, perhaps a consequence of the increased secretion by the liver of apoB particles in FH. Tendon xanthoma involving the extensor tendons of the fingers, elbows, knees, and especially the Achilles tendons, are present in 75% of patients and are hallmarks of diagnosis (Figure 3.30 and Figure 3.31). Clinical events are not common before the 4th decade; however, by the 5th decade, roughly 50% of men are symptomatic. Disease onset is typically later in women. A diagnostic score chart to calculate the probability of FH is available (www.leefh.nl) or the Simon Broome criteria may be used. Hypothyroidism, nephrotic syndrome, and obstructive liver disease should be excluded.

3.3.1.2 Homozygous FH (HOFH)

Homozygous FH (HoFH) occurs in approximately 1 in 1 million persons worldwide. Homozygous FH results from two defective alleles in the gene for the LDL receptor. Compound heterozygotes make up the large majority.

Clinical Diagnosis

ApoB is usually > 2.0 g/ l; total cholesterol levels are usually ≥ 14 mmol/l and can be > 20 mmol/l. Planar or tuberous cutaneous xanthomata and tendon xanthoma are present in childhood. HoFH can be fatal in childhood. Critical aortic stenosis may develop in childhood. Carotid and femoral disease develop later in life and are usually not clinically significant. Why these arteries are less susceptible than the coronaries is not known and this interesting discordance in clinical expression has unfortunately received little attention. HoFH is gender neutral with no major difference in prognosis between men and women. A careful family history should be taken, and plasma apoB levels should be measured in the parents and other first-degree relatives of patients with HoFH. Molecular assays are available to define the mutations in the LDL receptor by DNA sequencing but are not clinically required. Prognosis is driven by the level of LDL, not the molecular basis for the elevated level of LDL.

Genetic Causes

The most common mutations present in patients with FH are in the LDL receptor. The gene for the LDL receptor is present on the short arm of chromosome 19 and is made up of 18 exons, which span 45 kb and encode a single chain glycoprotein of 839 amino acids. More than 1000 functionally significant mutations in the LDL receptor have been described. The pathophysiology of FH due to defective function of an LDL receptor has been described in Chapter 1, section 1.4.4 and Figure 1.25.

3.3.1.3 Familial Defective ApoB100

Pathophysiology
Patients with familial defective apoB100 (FDB) synthesize an abnormal apoB100, most commonly due to a substitution of glutamine for arginine at position 3500, although other rarer mutations have been reported.[147-149] This abnormal apoB100 cannot bind appropriately to a normal LDL receptor. Thus, in contrast with FH, it is the ligand, apoB, not the LDL receptor, which is abnormal (Figure 3.28 en 3.29). FDB is an autosomal dominant disorder and heterozygotes present with mild or moderate HyperapoB due to a mild or moderate increase in the number of LDL particles. In heterozygotes, approximately half the LDL particles contain a normal apoB molecule while the other half of the LDL particles are enveloped by abnormal apoB molecules. LDL particles with the abnormal apoB are removed much more slowly from plasma than the normal LDL particles with a consequent increase in LDL particle number. The frequency of FDB has been stated to be 0.1% in the general population but this may be an overestimate, except in populations with significant numbers of individuals of German descent where the frequency can be as high as 1 in 1000. The hyperlipidemia that results is, as expected, characterized by an increased LDL cholesterol and plasma apoB with a normal triglyceride.

Clinical Diagnosis
Patients with FDB cannot be clinically distinguished from patients with HeFH, although patients with FDB tend to have lower plasma levels of apoB and LDL-C than FH heterozygotes. Tendon xanthomas and an increased incidence of premature CVD are common features.

3.3.1.4 PCSK9 Gain of Function
PCSK9 promotes degradation of the LDL receptor in the liver, thus reducing the clearance of circulating LDL particles.[150] A gain of function mutation can significantly reduce the number of LDL receptors at the cell surface producing a clinical syndrome that resembles severe HeFH with high apoB and LDL-C (Figure 3.28 en 3.29). Of interest, other individuals have been identified in whom genetic variants of PCSK9 impair its function, increasing LDL catabolism, resulting in low LDL cholesterol levels and a reduced risk of CAD.[151] Patients with PCSK-9 gain of function cannot be clinically distinguished from patients with HeFH or FDB. Thus, PCSK-9 gain of function is also characterized by HyperapoB due to an elevated LDL particle number and elevated plasma LDL-C levels with normal triglycerides, tendon xanthomas, and an increased incidence of premature CVD.

3.3.1.5 Polygenic Familial Hypercholesterolemia

These patients have the clinical syndrome of HeFH due to defective function of the LDL-receptor pathway. However, no single gene is responsible.[152] The clinical consequences relate to the phenotype not the genotype. That is, arterial damage relates to the markedly elevated level of LDL regardless of the cause. Thus, the indication for treatment and the modalities of treatment are the same as in the monogenic disorders of the LDL-receptor pathway. The importance of this finding is that family screening strategies should be based on the identification of an individual with the severe hypercholesterolemic phenotype.

3.3.1.6 Autosomal-Recessive Hypercholesterolemia (ARH)

Pathophysiology

ARH, a rare disorder (except in patients from Sardinia, Italy and the Middle East) is due to mutations in the gene for a putative adaptor protein called ARH (also called LDLR adaptor protein), which is involved in the internalization of LDL from the cell surface by endocytosis once it has bound to its receptor.[153,154]

Clinical Diagnosis

ARH clinically resembles HoFH and is therefore characterized by extremely high apoB and LDL-C, tendon xanthomas, and premature CVD. The level of LDL tends to be intermediate between the levels seen in FH homozygotes and FH heterozygotes.

3.3.2 Treatment of the Severe Hypercholesterolemic Phenotypes

Patients with severe hypercholesterolemic phenotypes should be aggressively treated to lower plasma levels of LDL-C and apoB. Dietary therapy will not reduce apoB and/or LDL-C to target levels in most patients. Statins are the primary agent but combination drug therapy with the addition of a cholesterol absorption inhibitor is frequently required. Often treatment targets cannot be reached but 50% reduction in apoB should be the minimum achieved.

Patients who cannot be adequately controlled on combination drug therapy may be candidates for selective LDL apheresis. MTP inhibitor (lomitapide) and anti-apoB RNA antisense therapy to reduce apoB secretion (mipomersen) will reduce apoB secretion and can substantially reduce plasma LDL-C and apoB. Both are now available in the US although mipomersen has not yet been approved in Europe. The PCSK-9 inhibitors, which are designed to enhance LDL-receptor function by blocking PCSK-9 binding to the LDL receptors, are an even more promising option. These are now undergoing clinical trials and may soon become available (*see also Table 4.6 in Chapter 4*).

3.3.3 Polygenic Hypercholesterolemia

Clinical diagnosis

Polygenic hypercholesterolemia is characterized by mild to moderate hypercholesterolemia due to elevated LDL-C with a normal plasma level of triglycerides in the absence of secondary causes of hypercholesterolemia. However, only a portion of the total number of patients with polygenic hypercholesterolemia, have an elevated apoB. Those with an elevated LDL C and an elevated apoB are at increased risk of CVD whereas those with an elevated LDL C but normal apoB – often healthy young women – are not (*section 2.2 – see normoapoB normoTG*).

Plasma LDL-C and apoB levels are generally not as elevated as they are in FH and FDB. Family studies are useful to differentiate polygenic hypercholesterolemia from the single-gene disorders; half of the first-degree relatives of patients with FH and FDB are hypercholesterolemic whereas < 10% of first-degree relatives of patients with polygenic hypercholesterolemia have hypercholesterolemia.

Treatment

Treatment of polygenic hypercholesterolemia with elevated apoB is identical to that of other forms of hyperapoB – low-cholesterol, low-fat diet is recommended and if targets are not reached, lipid-lowering drug therapy. Statins should be the primary therapy to reduce apoB to the appropriate target level, with ezetimibe added if necessary to reach the appropriate apoB target level (apoB < 0.75 g/L in high risk and < 0.65 g/l in very high risk patients). Rarely, a third drug, such as bile acid sequestrant or nicotinic acid, is needed to reduce apoB to target levels.

3.3.4 CYP7A1 Deficiency

Pathophysiology

Cholesterol 7 alpha-hydroxylase, also known as cholesterol 7 alpha-monooxygenase or cytochrome P450 7A1 (CYP7A1), is the rate-limiting enzyme in the production of bile acids from cholesterol and therefore in the catabolism of cholesterol. Decreased CYP7A1 levels, due to mutations in the gene, may lead to HyperapoB and high LDL-C. Some subjects who were homozygous for mutations in the CYP7A1 gene also had elevated plasma triglyceride levels. Premature coronary and peripheral vascular disease have been reported in homozygous patients. Individuals heterozygous for the mutations are also hyperlipidemic, indicating that this is a co-dominant disorder.

Treatment

As might be anticipated, these patients are resistant to statins. In principle, agents that reduce cholesterol absorption, such as ezetimibe, should be helpful.[66]

3.3.5 Hypoalphalipoproteinemia

Pathophysiology

A low plasma HDL-C (the alpha lipoprotein) is referred to as hypoalphalipoproteinemia and accelerated catabolism of HDL appears to be the primary metabolic abnormality responsible for this syndrome. Low HDL-C may be familial with an autosomal dominant pattern. However, in some patients with low HDL-C and normal lipids, apoB and LDL-C may be elevated.[66] In these patients, the high apoB may be secondary to the low HDL-C. The sequence may be as follows: HDL removes cholesterol from the liver as well as from peripheral tissues. If removal of cholesterol by HDL is defective, more cholesterol must be secreted with apoB particles to maintain hepatic cholesterol homeostasis. The increased secretion of VLDL particles leads to increased production of LDL particles and therefore elevated plasma apoB.

Clinical Diagnosis

Primary hypoalphalipoproteinemia is defined as a plasma HDL-C level below the tenth percentile in the setting of relatively normal cholesterol and triglyceride levels; no apparent secondary causes of low plasma HDL-C such as hypertriglyceridemia and no clinical signs of lecithin-cholesterol acyltransferase (LCAT) deficiency or Tangier disease. Several kindreds with primary hypoalphalipoproteinemia have been described in association with an increased incidence of premature CAD, although this is not an invariant association. Indeed, no definitive causal relation has been established.

Treatment

Patients with hypoalphalipoproteinemia and high apoB should be treated to lower plasma levels of apoB. Statins are the appropriate pharmacological therapy.

3.3.6 Cholesteryl Ester Storage Disease (CESD)

Pathophysiology

CESD is an autosomal recessive disorder due to defective function of lysosomal acid lipase, the enzyme responsible for lysosomal hydrolysis of cholesterol ester.[155,156] Hepatomegaly with increased cholesterol ester mass results. Cholesterol synthesis is upregulated because normal regulatory control from cholesterol released from the lysosome is diminished or absent. This results in increased hepatic apoB secretion, which produces the elevated plasma LDL-C and apoB.

Treatment

Statin therapy is the preferred therapy in this rare disorder. Plasma LDL is reduced as is the mass of cholesterol ester in the liver.

3.3.7 Hypercholesterolemic NormoapoB Phenotype

A critical and as yet unappreciated reason for measuring apoB rather than relying entirely on LDL-C or even non-HDL-C is that an important portion of subjects with an elevated LDL-C or non-HDL-C – approximately 1 in 4 – have a normal apoB. That is, these subjects have cholesterol-enriched LDL with the result that cholesterol levels are high but atherogenic particle number is not. Typically these subjects with hypercholesterolemic NormoapoB (HyperC NormoapoB) do not have the other features associated with FCH such as hypertriglyceridemia, hypertension and dysglycemia.

The distinction is critical to make because subjects with HyperC NormoapoB are not at increased cardiovascular risk. If only their LDL-C or non-HDL-C is measured, statin therapy might be given and this would be inappropriate. Even if pharmacological therapy is not initiated, raising concern as to whether a major risk factor is present is also inappropriate and could be psychologically harmful.

4. Secondary ApoB Dyslipoproteinemias

In this chapter, we will review the pathophysiology, clinical features, diagnostic criteria and treatment of the secondary apoB dyslipoproteinemias as classified by the apoB diagnostic algorithm.

Overview of the secondary apoB dyslipoproteinemias

- Diabetes Mellitus type 2 / Metabolic syndrome / Abdominal obesity (par. 4.2, page 117)
- Polycystic ovary syndrome (par. 4.3, page 124)
- Glucocorticoids (par. 4.4, page 124)
- Antipsychotic drugs (par. 4.5, page 125)
- Systemic lupus erythematosus (par. 4.6, page 125)
- Nephrotic syndrome (par. 4.7, page 127)
- Hemodialysis (par. 4.8, page 128)
- Continuous ambulatory peritoneal dialysis (par. 4.9, page 128)
- End-stage renal disease (par. 4.10, page 129)
- Cholestasis (par. 4.11, page 129)
- Pregnancy 3rd term (par. 4.12, page 130)
- Alcohol (par. 4.13, page 131)
- Estrogens (par. 4.14, page 132)
- Hypothyroidism (par. 4.15, page 132)
- HIV (par. 4.16, page 133)
- Anabolic steroids (par. 4.17, page 134)

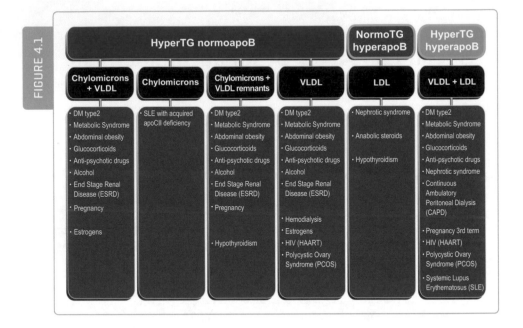

FIGURE 4.1

HyperTG normoapoB				NormoTG hyperapoB	HyperTG hyperapoB
Chylomicrons + VLDL	Chylomicrons	Chylomicrons + VLDL remnants	VLDL	LDL	VLDL + LDL
· DM type2 · Metabolic Syndrome · Abdominal obesity · Glucocorticoids · Anti-psychotic drugs · Alcohol · End Stage Renal Disease (ESRD) · Pregnancy · Estrogens	· SLE with acquired apoCII deficiency	· DM type2 · Metabolic Syndrome · Abdominal obesity · Glucocorticoids · Anti-psychotic drugs · Alcohol · End Stage Renal Disease (ESRD) · Pregnancy · Hypothyroidism	· DM type2 · Metabolic Syndrome · Abdominal obesity · Glucocorticoids · Anti-psychotic drugs · Alcohol · End Stage Renal Disease (ESRD) · Hemodialysis · Estrogens · HIV (HAART) · Polycystic Ovary Syndrome (PCOS)	· Nephrotic syndrome · Anabolic steroids · Hypothyroidism	· DM type2 · Metabolic Syndrome · Abdominal obesity · Glucocorticoids · Anti-psychotic drugs · Nephrotic syndrome · Continuous Ambulatory Peritoneal Dialysis (CAPD) · Pregnancy 3rd term · HIV (HAART) · Polycystic Ovary Syndrome (PCOS) · Systemic Lupus Erythematosus (SLE)

4.1 Introduction

The apoB dyslipoproteinemias are, not surprisingly, frequently the consequences of other disorders (see fly leaf of this book). They are secondary manifestations of the primary disorder. Accordingly, identifying and treating the primary abnormality is always the primary therapeutic maneuver. That diabetes, insulin resistance, and the metabolic syndrome are often associated with dyslipoproteinemia is well known. Less well appreciated is how diverse the secondary consequences of the same primary abnormality can be. Thus, the manifestations of dyslipoproteinemia in patients with diabetes may range from markedly increased chylomicron particle number to elevated VLDL particle number but normal LDL particle number to increased chylomicron and VLDL remnant particle number to elevated VLDL and LDL particle number. Why there is such a range of secondary manifestations for what is generally considered one disorder, such as diabetes mellitus, is one of the most intriguing but unanswered questions in lipidology. Recognizing their individual characteristics, however, is key to instituting appropriate therapy. Accordingly, in this chapter, we discuss the different apoB phenotypes that are associated with a range of primary disorders with comments on pathophysiology, clinical characteristics, and treatment.

4.2 Type 2 Diabetes Mellitus, Metabolic Syndrome, Abdominal Obesity

Hypertriglyceridemia and low HDL-C are the typical lipid abnormalities in patients who are overweight or obese or who have DM2 or who have the metabolic syndrome whereas levels of LDL-C, characteristically, are normal in all of these. In a lipid-driven approach attention, naturally, has focused on VLDL and HDL with the result that the atherogenic risk posed by the elevated levels of cholesterol-depleted LDL particles has not been appreciated. The apoB algorithm allows the different phenotypes of hyper-triglyceridemia to be distinguished and the total number of atherogenic particles to be quantitated. As it turns out, elevation of atherogenic apoB particle number – Hyper-apoB – is the commonest abnormality in patients with DM2 or metabolic syndrome or abdominal obesity and, therefore, an increased number of LDL particles is the dominant proatherogenic lipoprotein abnormality, a finding that was missed by conventional lipid tests, which emphasized VLDL and HDL and deemphasized LDL (*see Figure 1.12*).[31,157] Not only does apoB predict the risk of CVD in patients with type 1[158] and type 2 diabetes[159-161] but apoB deposition may be involved in the progression of the micro-vascular disease responsible for diabetic nephropathy[162] and diabetic retinopathy.[163] That said, other abnormalities also contribute to the increased risk of diabetic nephropathy and CVD in patients with diabetes – that is to both the risk of microvascular as well as macrovascular disease. These may include alterations in LDL such as glycation and alterations in the glycosaminoglycans, the ground substance of the arterial wall.[164] Finally there is the fascinating possibility that HyperapoB may contribute to the pathogenesis of diabetes, perhaps by pancreatic injury due to excessive uptake of LDL particles.[165,166] With regard to therapy, except for those with remnant lipoprotein dis-order, apoB should be the target of LDL-lowering therapy. Non-HDL-C and LDL-C often do not accurately reflect the levels of apoB and therefore are not adequate targets.[167]

We will now discuss the 4 different apoB phenotypes that can be present in subjects with DM2, the metabolic syndrome or abdominal obesity (*Figure 4.1*).

4.2.1 HyperTG HyperapoB: Increased VLDL and LDL Lipoprotein Particles

Pathophysiology of Increased VLDL and LDL Particle Number
The most frequently observed atherogenic dyslipoproteinemia in overweight or obese patients with DM2 or metabolic syndrome is the HyperTG HyperapoB phenotype, which is defined as an increased number of VLDL and LDL particles. HDL-C is often low as well (*Figure 4.2*). In *Figure 4.3* a general overview of the different mechanisms contributing to dyslipidemia are indicated. Increased flux of free fatty acids from adipocytes to hepatocytes results in increased synthesis and secretion of triglycerides

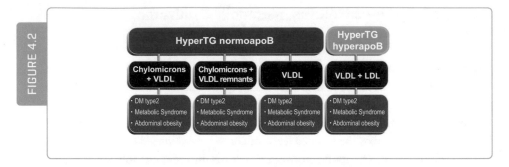

FIGURE 4.2

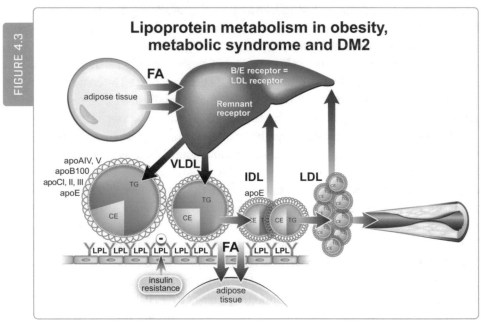

FIGURE 4.3

and cholesterol ester with the result that increased numbers of VLDL particles are secreted resulting in increased formation of LDL particles – thus the increased apoB. Hyperinsulinemia, due to insulin resistance in obesity, promotes fatty acid and cholesterol synthesis in the liver, which adds to the tendency to increased VLDL production and secretion of VLDL particles. VLDL catabolism may be impaired due to decreased LPL activity, which can be associated with insulin resistance. Increased apoCIII may contribute both to increased synthesis and decreased clearance of triglyceride (*see Figure 1.15*). ApoCIII may also increase the conversion of VLDL particles to LDL particles.[7] Increased CETP activity also contributes to the atherogenic lipoprotein phenotype characterized by high apoB, low HDL-C, small, cholesterol depleted LDL, high triglycerides with relatively cholesterol-rich VLDL particles (*see Figure 1.12*).

Clinical Diagnosis

No diagnostic stigmata of high VLDL and LDL are present on physical examination.

Treatment

Individuals with obesity, metabolic syndrome, DM2 and increased VLDL and LDL (HyperTG HyperapoB) should be treated aggressively due to their significantly increased risk of premature CVD (Table 4.1) . Weight loss is a difficult but necessary objective and weight loss and aerobic exercise can have beneficial effects on the lipid profile. However, the great majority will require lipid-lowering drug therapy to reduce atherogenic apoB lipoprotein levels to the recommended range (< 0.75 g/l for high-risk and < 0.65 g/l for very high-risk patients) necessary to reduce the high risk of CVD. Note apoB, not triglycerides, are the primary target of therapy. Statins are effective in this condition, but many patients will need a second drug such as a cholesterol absorption inhibitor (ezetimibe) for optimal control of apoB levels. Such agents are also necessary for statin-intolerant patients. The IMPROVE-IT study demonstrated additional clinical benefit with ezetimibe plus statin and this result supports its use in the appropriate clinical settings. Pharmacological therapy with fibrates added to statins has been suggested to reduce triglycerides and increase HDL-C in very high-risk patients. However, clinical trial results have not supported this combination, albeit the subjects were not selected for this phenotype.

Table 4.1

Steps in treatment	HyperTG HyperapoB (increased VLDL and LDL particles)
General measures including lifestyle intervention and check for / treat other secondary or primary causes	Weight loss, exercise, stop smoking, stop alcohol, decrease saturated fat and simple carbohydrates intake
Risk of CVD	++(+)
Treatment to prevent CVD	1. statins
	2. ezetimibe
Targets to prevent CVD	apoB < 0.75 g/l in moderate and high risk
	apoB < 0.65 g/l in very high risk
Risk of pancreatitis	—

4.2.2 HyperTG NormoapoB: Increased VLDL Lipoprotein Particles

Pathophysiology of High VLDL
If triglyceride synthesis and secretion are increased but VLDL apoB secretion is normal, the number of LDL particles will be normal and therefore total plasma apoB will be 'normal' (that is < 1.20 g/l) in the face of an elevated plasma triglyceride (≥ 1.5 mmol/l). If so, the VLDL particles are likely to be triglyceride enriched. Alternatively, this phenotype may be due to a decreased clearance rate of VLDL particles coupled to a normal production rate, as could occur with primary or secondary impairment of LPL activity (*Chapter 3, section 3.1.4*).

Clinical Diagnosis
No diagnostic stigmata attributable to high VLDL are present on physical examination.

Treatment
Because the number of atherogenic particles is not markedly increased (apoB < 1.20 g/l), the atherogenic risk of this dyslipoproteinemia is not markedly increased (*Table 4.2*). But there is nothing magic in the dividing line of 1.20 g/l. Cardiovascular risk rises exponentially as the level of apoB increases and therefore the higher the apoB, the higher the risk. Just as importantly, it is the apoB that is the issue, not the triglycerides since there is no evidence that lowering triglycerides improves clinical outcome. In patients with other high-risk abnormalities, such as DM2, pharmacological therapy would be indicated to lower apoB. If so, statins should be the primary therapy to reduce apoB to the appropriate target level with ezetimibe added if necessary to reach the appropriate apoB target level (apoB < 0.75 g/l in high-risk and < 0.65 g/l in very high-risk patients).

Table 4.2

Steps in treatment	HyperTG NormoapoB (increased VLDL particles)
General measures including lifestyle intervention and check for / treat other secondary or primary causes	Weight loss, exercise, stop smoking, stop alcohol, decrease saturated fat and simple carbohydrates intake
Risk of CVD	+/- depending on associated high-risk conditions ie DM2 etc
Treatment to prevent CVD	1. statins
	2. ezetimibe
Targets to prevent CVD	apoB < 0.75 g/l in moderate and high risk
	apoB < 0.65 g/l in very high risk
Risk of pancreatitis	—

Ezetimibe can be used in patients who do not tolerate statins. As increased triglyceride levels are the main lipid presentation of this phenotype, clinicians might consider fibrates. However, while fibrates lower triglyceride levels, they only modestly lower the number of atherogenic apoB particles and there is insufficient randomized clinical trial evidence to justify their use in this phenotype.

4.2.3 HyperTG NormoapoB: Increased Chylomicron and VLDL Lipoprotein Particles

Pathophysiology of Excess Chylomicron and VLDL
In some patients with obesity, especially those with an associated genetic defect in lipid metabolism (see Chapter 3, section 3.1.2), serum triglycerides can be extremely elevated. Obesity, particularly abdominal obesity, can lead to increased production of VLDL due to increased flux of fatty acids to the liver. If partial LPL deficiency were also present, the combination might result in the phenotype of an increased number of triglyceride-rich VLDL and chylomicron particles.

Clinical Consequences
Patients with severe hypertriglyceridemia due to chylomicrons and VLDL particles may present with eruptive xanthomata (Figure 3.6) and their plasma may appear milky (Figure 3.9). If chylomicron and VLDL particle numbers are increased sufficiently, pancreatitis may occur. In such patients, plasma triglycerides will generally be > 10 mmol/l. Plasma apoB is only occasionally elevated above the 75th percentile (i.e. > 1.20 g/l); in these patients, lowering of apoB is indicated. For those with intermediate apoB levels (0.75-1.20 g/l), the decision to institute apoB-lowering therapy should be based on the associated clinical characteristics of the patient.

Treatment
In those with severe hypertriglyceridemia who are at risk of pancreatitis, dietary total fat intake should be reduced, acutely and profoundly (Table 4.3). Other secondary or primary causes should be identified and, if present, treated. Treatment with fibrates may be helpful in these patients as partial LPL activity is likely present. Nicotinic acid or long-chain n-3 polyunsaturated fatty acids (PUFAs) remain an option but the clinical trial evidence is lacking. Whether apoB-lowering therapy with statins is indicated depends on the level of apoB and the clinical circumstances. Thus, patients with increased cardiovascular risk because of the presence of DM2 or a history of CVD will require apoB-lowering therapy to target apoB levels < 0.65 g/l.

Table 4.3

Steps in treatment	HyperTG NormoapoB (increased chylomicron and VLDL particles)
General measures including lifestyle intervention and check for / treat other secondary or primary causes	- fasting for > 24 hours - IV fluids if necessary - insulin drip - dietary fat restriction 15 g/d - followed by low fat diet - no alcohol, weight loss, treat diabetes
Risk of CVD	Depends on apoB and associated high risk conditions
Treatment to prevent CVD	statins
Targets to prevent CVD	apoB < 0.75 g/l in moderate and high risk apoB < 0.65 g/l in very high risk
Risk of pancreatitis	++
Treatment to prevent pancreatitis	1. fibrates
	2. long chain n-3 PUFA
	3. nicotinic acid
Target to prevent pancreatitis	TG < 5 mmol/l

4.2.4 HyperTG NormoapoB: Increased Chylomicron and VLDL Remnant Lipoprotein particles

Pathophysiology of Chylomicron and VLDL Remnants – Remnant Lipoprotein Disorder

Familial dysbetalipoproteinemia (FDBL) or remnant lipoprotein disorder may become evident in patients with obesity, metabolic syndrome or DM2. FDBL is characterized by markedly increased numbers of chylomicron and VLDL remnants (Chapter 3, section 3.1.3). However, homozygosity of apoE2/E2 alleles is not sufficient to produce the full clinical syndrome. Only 1 in 50 to 1 in 100 of apoE2 homozygotes have the clinical profile of FDBL. There is also evidence that most patients with FDBL are not apoE2/E2. Given that FDBL is only present in a small minority of apoE2 homozygotes, some additional provoking factor must be present to produce the full clinical syndrome. This second abnormality is generally one that increases fatty acid flux to the liver with the result that VLDL apoB production increases. The most common precipitating factors are a high-fat diet, DM2, obesity and the metabolic syndrome. Furthermore, hypothyroidism, renal disease, estrogen deficiency, alcohol use, or certain drugs may be involved.

Clinical Diagnosis

Chylomicron and VLDL remnants are extremely atherogenic lipoprotein particles and peripheral vascular disease is a major clinical feature in these patients as well as CAD. Think of remnant lipoprotein disorder when tubero-eruptive and palmar xanthomas (*Figure 3.15 and 3.17*), premature CAD and peripheral vascular disease are found in obese patients with or without metabolic syndrome or DM2 (*FDBL, Chapter 3, section 3.1.3*).

Treatment

Since remnants are associated with markedly increased risk of premature CVD, this atherogenic apoB phenotype should be treated aggressively (*Table 4.4*). The first step is to treat the conditions that precipitate the expression of the phenotype, such as obesity, DM2, metabolic syndrome, significant alcohol intake and hypothyroidism. Weight reduction is recommended. Alcohol intake should be curtailed and estrogen treatment stopped. Pharmacological treatment is aimed at decreasing the number of atherogenic remnant particles. In this instance, risk would be severely underestimated if total plasma apoB were relied on. Treatment should aim at normal levels of cholesterol (< 5 mmol/l) and triglyceride (< 2 mmol/l) and apoB levels < 0.65 g/l. Patients with remnant lipoprotein disorder may respond well to fibrates as well as statins or even nicotinic acid. Occasionally, combination drug therapy is required.

Table 4.4

Steps in treatment	HyperTG NormoapoB (increased chylomicron and VLDL remnant particles)
General measures including lifestyle intervention and check for / treat other secondary or primary causes	Stop smoking, exercise, diet, stop alcohol, check medication ie stop estrogens, check for hypothyroidism, treat DM etc.
Risk of CVD	+++
Treatment to prevent CVD	1. statins
	2. fibrates
	3. Nicotinic acid
Targets to prevent CVD	apoB < 0.65 g/l +
	total cholesterol < 5 mmol/l +
	TG < 2 mmol/l
Risk of pancreatitis	—

4.3 Polycystic Ovary Syndrome (PCOS)

Oligomenorrhea or anovulation, polycystic ovaries on pelvic ultrasonography, hyper-androgenism and infertility are the key endocrine features of PCOS. Affected women may also have obesity and insulin resistance. Hypertriglyceridemia and low HDL-C are therefore the typical lipid abnormalities in patients with PCOS whereas LDL-C levels, characteristically, are normal. By measuring apoB, total cholesterol and triglycerides and applying the ApoB algorithm, increased numbers of atherogenic cholesterol-depleted LDL particles (HyperTG HyperapoB) can be distinguished from the presence of HyperTG NormoapoB reflecting the presence of increased VLDL particles.

HyperTG HyperapoB due to VLDL+ LDL or HyperTG-NormoApoB due to VLDL
The most frequently observed dyslipoproteinemia in obese patients with PCOS is the HyperTG HyperapoB phenotype. HDL-C is often low as well.[168,169] In non-obese women, apoB tends to be normal and impaired cholesterol efflux from peripheral cells has been described.[170] Increased flux of free fatty acids from adipocytes to hepatocytes results in increased synthesis and secretion of VLDL particles with increased formation of LDL particles, which produces the increased apoB. Hyperinsulinemia due to insulin resistance promotes fatty acid and cholesterol synthesis in the liver, which adds to the tendency to increased VLDL production and secretion of VLDL particles. Also VLDL catabolism may be impaired due to decreased LPL activity, which can be associated with insulin resistance (Figure 4.3). Approximately 50% of women with PCOS also suffer from the metabolic syndrome.

The treatment of high VLDL and LDL or isolated high VLDL are indicated above and in Chapter 3 and presented in Table 4.1 and 4.2.

4.4 Glucocorticoids

Glucocorticoids can produce a variety of abnormalities including HyperTG HyperapoB due to VLDL+LDL and HyperTG NormoapoB due to chylomicrons + VLDL particles, VLDL + chylomicron remnants or VLDL (Figure 4.1). By measuring only lipids, the four different types of hypertriglyceridemia – VLDL + LDL, VLDL, chylomicron + VLDL remnants and chylomicron + VLDL – cannot be easily and accurately distinguished. Measuring apoB, cholesterol and triglyceride not only allows these four phenotypes to be identified but also allows increased numbers of cholesterol-depleted LDL particles to be distinguished from increased numbers of remnant particles. All can be distinguished by the apoB algorithm.

Excess glucocorticoids can produce cervical and abdominal obesity with typical striae, hirsutism and hypertension. Obesity results in increased flux of free fatty acids from adipocytes to hepatocytes resulting in increased synthesis and secretion of VLDL particles with increased formation of LDL particles, which produces the increased apoB. Hyperinsulinemia, due to insulin resistance associated with glucocorticoid use, promotes fatty acid and cholesterol synthesis in the liver, which adds to the tendency to increased VLDL production and section of VLDL particles. Also VLDL catabolism may be impaired due to decreased LPL activity, which can be associated with insulin resistance (Figure 4.3).

In some patients treated with glucocorticoids, especially those with a genetic defect in lipid metabolism (see Chapter 3, section 3.1.3), serum triglycerides can be extremely elevated. If partial LPL deficiency were also present, the combination might result in the phenotype of an increased number of triglyceride-rich VLDL and chylomicron particles. Then patients may present with eruptive xanthomata (Figure 3.6) and plasma may appear milky (Figure 3.9, see Familial Hyperchylomicronemia – section 3.1.1 and section 3.1.2).

If chylomicron and VLDL particle numbers are increased sufficiently, pancreatitis may occur. Finally, remnant lipoprotein disorder may become evident in patients treated with corticosteroids. Think of this diagnosis when tubero-eruptive (Figure 3.15) and palmar xanthomas (Figure 3.17), premature coronary disease and peripheral vascular disease are found in a patient treated with corticosteroids (see Chapter 3, section 3.1.3).

The treatment of hyperTG hyperapoB due to VLDL+LDL and HyperTG NormoapoB due to chylomicrons + VLDL particles, VLDL + chylomicron remnants or VLDL are indicated above and in Chapter 3 and presented in Table 4.1, 4.2, 4.3 and 4.4.

4.5 Antipsychotic Drugs

Hypertriglyceridemia with or without hypercholesterolemia and low HDL-C are typical lipid abnormalities in patients treated with antipsychotic agents. By measuring apoB, total cholesterol and triglycerides and applying the apoB algorithm, it is now possible to distinguish HyperTG HyperapoB due to presence of VLDL and LDL or HyperTG NormoapoB due to VLDL, chylomicron and VLDL particles or chylomicron and VLDL remnants (Figure 4.1).

HyperTG HyperapoB due to LDL and VLDL is the typical lipoprotein abnormality in subjects using antipsychotic drugs. Antipsychotics have been associated with weight gain, obesity, which can produce increased flux of free fatty acids from adipocytes to hepatocytes resulting in increased synthesis and secretion of VLDL particles with increased formation of LDL particles, which produces the HyperapoB HyperTG phenotype (Figure 4.3).

HyperTG NormoapoB due to remnant lipoprotein disorder and/or increased chylo-microns and VLDL have also been described. The familial dysbetalipoproteinemia phenotype (FDBL) may become evident in patients treated with antipsychotic agents. Think of FDBL when tubero-eruptive (*Figure 3.15*) and palmar xanthomas (*Figure 3.17*), premature CAD and peripheral vascular disease are found in patients treated with antipsychotic drugs (*see Chapter 3, section 3.1.3*).

In some patients treated with antipsychotic agents, especially those with a genetic defect in lipid metabolism (*see Chapter 3*), serum triglycerides can be extremely elevated. Obesity, particularly abdominal obesity, can lead to increased production of VLDL due to increased flux of fatty acids to the liver. If partial LPL deficiency were also present, the combination might result in the phenotype of an increased number of triglyceride-rich VLDL and chylomicron particles. All these apoB phenotypes can be distinguished by the apoB algorithm and their treatments have been described above and presented in *Table 4.1, 4.2, 4.3, 4.4*.

4.6 Systemic Lupus Erythematosus

Hypertriglyceridemia, hypercholesterolemia and low HDL-C are the typical lipid ab-normalities in patients with SLE. By measuring apoB, total cholesterol and triglycerides one can distinguish the most common dyslipoproteinemia in patients with SLE - Hyper-apoB HyperTG due to the presence of LDL and VLDL whereas hyperTG NormoapoB due to the excess of chylomicrons is uncommon.

The triglyceride within chylomicrons is normally rapidly hydrolyzed by lipoprotein lipase (LPL) in adipose tissue and skeletal muscle and the remnant particle that is produced, which contains some of the original triglyceride and all of the original cholesterol, is then rapidly removed by the liver (*Chapter 1, section 1.1.3*). In SLE, marked hyperchylomicronemia may occur due to an antibody to apoCII, that precludes activation of LPL or due to an antibody to LPL itself. The risk of pancreatitis becomes substantial when plasma triglyceride levels are more than 10 mmol/l. Other major clinical features include: eruptive xanthomata, small, yellowish-white papules, often in clusters on the back, buttocks, and extensor surfaces of the arms and legs (*Figure 3.6*); lipaemia retinalis (on fundoscopic examination the retinal blood vessels are opalescent (*Figure 3.7 and 3.8*)); and hepatosplenomegaly due to the uptake of circulating chylo-microns by reticuloendothelial cells in the liver and spleen. A blood sample may appear pale and the serum milky (*Figure 3.9*). Pseudohyponatremia may be present.

Their treatment is described in *Table 4.1* for high VLDL and LDL and in *Table 4.5* for high chylomicrons.

Table 4.5

Steps in treatment	HyperTG NormoapoB (increased chylomicron particles)
General measures including lifestyle intervention and check for / treat other secondary or primary causes	- fasting for > 24 hours. - IV fluids - insulin drip - plasmapharesis if critically ill - dietary fat restriction 15 g/d - followed by low fat diet - no alcohol, weight loss, treat DM
Risk of CVD	—
Treatment to prevent CVD	—
Targets to prevent CVD	—
Risk of pancreatitis	+++
Treatment to prevent pancreatitis	1. low fat diet
	2. fibrates
	3. medium chain triglycerides
Target to prevent pancreatitis	TG < 5 mmol/l

4.7 Nephrotic Syndrome

Hypercholesterolemia with or without hypertriglyceridemia and low HDL C – that is, HyperTG HyperapoB due to VLDL and LDL and NormoTG HyperapoB due to LDL – are the typical apoB dyslipoprotcincmias abnormalities in patients with the nephrotic syndrome. Increased apoB secretion is the primary abnormality producing the elevated apoB. Reductions in LDL receptor activity might perhaps contribute due to higher PCSK9 levels. Multiple contributors for this include increased cholesterol synthesis, increased fatty acid flux to the liver, and reduced albumin. ApoB should be the target of treatment as described in Chapter 6. Treatment of the nephrotic syndrome is the primary objective. A variety of treatments have been reported depending on the cause and age of the subject. In addition to steroids, these include alkylating agents, anticalcineurin agents and humanized anti-CD20 monoclonal antibody. High-quality studies documenting the outcome of statin LDL-lowering therapy have not been published. LDL apheresis has been applied in occasional extreme cases. The argument has been made that intensive treatment of the lipid abnormality may improve the underlying disorder or at least improve the sensitivity of the underlying disorder to immunosuppressive therapy.

Both increased LDL (NormoTG HyperapoB) (Table 4.6) and increased VLDL and LDL (HyperTG HyperapoB (Table 4.1)) in patients with the nephrotic syndrome should be

Table 4.6

Steps in treatment	NormoTG HyperapoB (increased LDL particles)
General measures including lifestyle intervention and check for / treat other secondary or primary causes	Weight loss, exercise, stop smoking, stop alcohol, decrease saturated fat and simple carbohydrates intake
Risk of CVD	+++
Treatment to prevent CVD	1. statins
	2. ezetimibe
	3. In Severe Hypercholesterolemic Phenotype: lipoprotein apheresis, PCSK-9 inhibitors, MTP inhibitors, antisense apoB
Targets to prevent CVD	apoB < 0.75 g/l in moderate & high risk
	apoB < 0.65 g/l in very high risk
Risk of pancreatitis	—

treated due to their presumably significantly increased risk of premature CVD. Effective treatment of the underlying renal disease usually normalizes the lipoprotein phenotype but in the interim these patients will require lipid-lowering drug therapy to reduce atherogenic apoB lipoprotein levels to the recommended range (< 0.75 g/l in high risk and < 0.65 g/l in very high risk patients) and to reduce the high risk of CVD. Statins are effective in this condition. A second agent such as a cholesterol absorption inhibitor may be required.[171]

4.8 Hemodialysis

Conventionally, hemodialysis is associated with mild hypertriglyceridemia. Increased VLDL is, by far, the most common cause. By measuring apoB, other hypertriglyceridemic phenotypes can be differentiated. Treatment is discussed above and presented in Table 4.2. The conjunctive use of ezetimibe with statins is supported by the results of IMPROVE-IT and the SHARP trial.[172]

4.9 Continuous Ambulatory Peritoneal Dialysis

The most frequently observed dyslipoproteinemia in patients treated with CAPD is the HyperTG HyperapoB phenotype, due an increased number of VLDL and LDL particles. HDL-C is often low as well. Treatment of this disorder is discussed above and presented in *Table 4.1*. The glucose load in the dialysate appears to contribute to the pathophysiology and low glucose dialysates are associated with metabolic amelioration.[173] Statin therapy is the main stay of therapy but reducing the concentration of glucose in the dialysate is also helpful.[174,175]

4.10 Chronic Renal Disease and End-Stage Renal Disease (ESRD)

Conventionally, hypertriglyceridemia and low HDL-C are the typical lipid abnormalities in patients with ESRD whereas LDL-C levels, characteristically, are normal. Three different types of hypertriglyceridemia – VLDL, chylomicron + VLDL remnants and chylomicron + VLDL – can be easily and accurately distinguished by measuring ApoB, triglycerides and cholesterol and applying the apoB algorithm (*Figure 4.1*).

In some patients treated for ESRD, especially those with a genetic defect in lipid metabolism (*see Chapter 3, primary causes*), serum triglycerides can be extremely elevated due to chylomicron and VLDL particles. Also remnant lipoprotein disorder may become evident in patients with ESRD. Think of FDBL when tubero-eruptive (*Figure 3.15*) and palmar xanthomas (*Figure 3.17*), premature CAD and peripheral vascular disease are found in a patient with ESRD (*see Chapter 3, section 3.1.3*).

Treatment is discussed above and in Chapter 3 and presented in the tables in this chapter. A Cochrane review supports the use of statins in patients with chronic renal disease.[176] The addition of ezetimibe is supported by the results of the SHARP trial.[172]

It is less clear whether LDL-lowering therapy is beneficial in patients with ESRD who are receiving hemodialysis therapy. Other mechanisms of cardiac ischemia and injury than plaque rupture are likely to be more important in this group.[177]

4.11 Cholestasis Primary Biliary Cirrhosis

NormoapoB Elevated LDL-C

Conventionally, cholestasis or primary biliary cirrhosis is often associated with marked hypercholesterolemia, which is associated with a high LDL-C. However, such patients often have cholesterol-rich particles, which are not true LDL particles. That is why most of these patients with a high cholesterol have a normal apoB. Measuring apoB demonstrates that atherogenic risk due to LDL is not increased.[178]

Pathophysiology

The major pathway by which cholesterol is excreted from the body is via secretion into bile, either directly or after conversion to bile acids. In cholestasis, this pathway is blocked and cholesterol accumulates within hepatocytes, which secrete an atypical particle, which is made up of free cholesterol coupled with phospholipids. This lamellar particle is called LP-X .

Clinical Diagnosis

The LP-X particles can be deposited in skin folds, producing lesions resembling those seen in patients with FDBL. Planar and eruptive xanthomas can also be seen in patients with cholestasis.

4.12 Pregnancy

Marked hypertriglyceridemia and hypercholesterolemia may occur during pregnancy.[179] HDL-C concentrations initially increase and then fall in the third trimester. By measuring only lipids, the three most common phenotypes of hypertriglyceridemia – VLDL + LDL versus chylomicron + VLDL versus chylomicrons + VLDL remnants – cannot be easily and accurately distinguished. Measuring apoB not only allows these three phenotypes to be easily distinguished, but also allows increased numbers of cholesterol-depleted LDL particles to be distinguished from increased numbers of remnant particles. High triglyceride concentrations may provide maternal fuel while sparing glucose for the fetus.

The most frequently observed dyslipoproteinemia during pregnancy is the HyperTG HyperapoB phenotype, due an increased number of VLDL and LDL particles. Increased release of free fatty acids from adipocytes, increased hepatic lipase activity and reduced LPL activity may all contribute. Impaired glucose tolerance post-partum, even if transient, may signal future risk of atherogenic dyslipoproteinemia and increased cardiovascular risk.[180]

Remnant lipoprotein disorder (familial dysbetalipoproteinemia) may become evident in pregnant women. FDBL is characterized by markedly increased numbers of chylomicron and VLDL remnants (Chapter 3, section 3.1.3); Think of FDBL when tubero-eruptive (Figure 3.15) and palmar xanthomas (Figure 3.17) are found in pregnant women.

In some pregnant women, especially those with a genetic defect in lipid metabolism (see Chapter 3 primary causes), serum triglycerides can be extremely elevated. Furthermore, obesity, particularly abdominal obesity, can lead to further increased production of VLDL due to increased flux of fatty acids to the liver. If partial LPL deficiency were also present, the combination might result in the phenotype of an increased number of triglyceride-rich VLDL and chylomicron particles. Patients with severe hypertriglyceridemia due to chylomicrons and VLDL particles may present with eruptive xanthomata (*Figure 3.6*) and plasma may appear milky (*Figure 3.9*) (*see FHC, Chapter 3, section 3.1.1*). If chylomicron and VLDL particle numbers are increased sufficiently, pancreatitis may occur.

Treatment

Pharmacological treatment during pregnancy is not advised. Women who develop this phenotype during pregnancy may be more likely to develop it again later in life. Low-fat diets may be helpful. This would be yet another argument for abstinence of alcohol. Long-chain 3n-PUFAs remain an option.

4.13 Alcohol

Hypertriglyceridemia can occur in patients consuming excess alcohol whereas LDL-C levels, characteristically, are normal. HDL-C, by contrast, may be elevated. By measuring only lipids, the different types of hypertriglyceridemia – VLDL, chylomicron + VLDL remnants and chylomicron + VLDL – cannot be distinguished. Measuring apoB allows these three phenotypes to be identified (*Figure 4.1*).

Alcohol may produce hypertriglyceridemia by inhibiting hepatic fatty acid oxidation. The excess fatty acids may stimulate triglyceride synthesis and secretion. If triglyceride synthesis and secretion are increased but VLDL apoB secretion is normal, the number of LDL particles will be normal and therefore total plasma apoB will be 'normal' (that is < 1.20 g/l) in the face of an elevated plasma triglyceride ($\geq$ 1.5 mmol/l). The VLDL particles are likely to be triglyceride enriched and/or increased in number. Alternatively, a reduced rate of triglyceride hydrolysis of VLDL particles will produce the same phenotype (*Chapter 1, section 1.4*).

Remnant lipoprotein disorder may become evident in patients with excessive alcoholic intake. Think of remnant lipoprotein disorder when tubero-eruptive (*Figure 3.15*) and palmar xanthomas (*Figure 3.17*), premature CAD and peripheral vascular disease are found in patients drinking excessive alcohol (*Chapter 3, primary causes*).

In some patients who drink excess alcohol, especially those with a genetic defect in lipid metabolism (*see Chapter 3, primary causes*), serum triglycerides can be extremely elevated.

If treatment is clinically indicated, the approaches recommended – stratified by different lipoprotein particles present – are outlined above and presented in the tables in this chapter and in *Chapter 3*.

4.14 Estrogens

The clinical belief that estrogens reduced cardiovascular events was upended by randomized clinical trials, a finding that has been a bulwark of the belief in RCTs. Nevertheless the issue may be more complex than was generally suspected and it is now argued that estrogen therapy to treat the symptoms of estrogen deficiency in appropriate cases is not unreasonable[181,182] However, oral estrogen administration can be associated with elevated serum levels of both triglycerides and HDL-C. Measuring apoB, together with total cholesterol and triglycerides, allows you to identify whether the hypertriglyceridemia is due to increased VLDL or to increased VLDL + chylomicrons. By the same token, remnant lipoprotein disorder has been recognized in some women who have lost the capacity to secrete estrogen.

Pathophysiology of High VLDL

If triglyceride synthesis and secretion are increased but VLDL apoB secretion is normal, the number of LDL particles will be normal and therefore total plasma apoB will be 'normal' (that is < 1.20 g/l) in the face of an elevated plasma triglyceride ($\geq$ 1.5 mmol/l). The VLDL particles are likely to be triglyceride enriched and/or increased in number. Alternatively, a reduced rate of triglyceride hydrolysis of VLDL particles will produce the same phenotype (*Chapter 1, section 1.2.2*).

In some patients treated with estrogens, especially those with a genetic defect in lipid metabolism (*Chapter 3, primary causes*), serum triglycerides can be extremely elevated. Obesity, particularly abdominal obesity, can lead to further increased production of VLDL due to increased flux of fatty acids to the liver. If partial LPL deficiency were also present, the combination might result in the phenotype of an increased number of triglyceride-rich VLDL and chylomicron particles.[183-188]

4.15 Hypothyroidism

Hypercholesterolemia with or without hypertriglyceridemia and low HDL-C can occur in hypothyroid patients, reflecting the presence of LDL or remnants. Hypothyroidism is divided into overt hypothyroidism (elevated thyroid-stimulating hormone (TSH); reduced thyroid hormone) and subclinical hypothyroidism (elevated TSH; normal thyroid hormone). Overt hypothyroidism needs to be treated with exogenous thyroid hormone. The effects of thyroid hormone on correcting the lipid abnormalities are not clear-cut. By measuring apoB the two different phenotypes, increased LDL particles or the presence of chylomicron + VLDL remnants, can be easily and accurately distinguished.

Pathophysiology of high LDL and high chylomicron and VLDL remnants

The primary mechanism for hypercholesterolemia in hypothyroidism is accumulation of LDL due to a reduction in the number of cell surface receptors for these particles, resulting in decreased catabolism of LDL. Thyroid hormone can also stimulate bile acid synthesis and reduce PCSK9. Reduction of these effects would contribute to increased levels of LDL through reduction of LDL-receptor activity or increase in apoB secretion.

Remnant lipoprotein disorder may become evident in patients with hypothyroidism. Think of familial dysbetalipoproteinemia when tubero-eruptive (Figure 3.15) and palmar xanthomas (Figure 3.17), premature CAD and peripheral vascular disease are found in a hypothyroid patient (Chapter 3, section 3.1.3).

Treatment

Individuals with hypothyroidism and increased LDL should be treated aggressively due to a significantly increased risk of premature CAD (Table 4.6). The first step is to treat the thyroid deficiency. Decreased dietary intake of saturated fat and simple carbohydrates, aerobic exercise, and weight loss can all have beneficial effects on the lipid profile. Patients with diabetes should be aggressively treated to maintain good glucose control. Statins should be the primary pharmacological agent to lower apoB.

4.16 HIV and HAART

Abnormalities of lipid metabolism were reported in the pre-HAART era in patients with advanced AIDS. HIV-infected patients tend to develop decreases in HDL-C followed by an increase in serum triglyceride levels and apoB prior to developing AIDS. Initiation of HAART could be associated with significant hypertriglyceridemia with or without elevated apoB, although the effect varied with the individual classes of antiretroviral drugs.[189-192]

The protease inhibitors appear to have the greatest negative impact on total cholesterol and triglyceride levels; however, even within this class, not all agents had an adverse effect on lipids. Hypertriglyceridemia with or without hypercholesterolemia and low HDL-C are the typical lipid abnormalities in patients with HIV on HAART therapy. By measuring apoB in combination with total cholesterol and triglycerides, you can easily distinguish which lipoprotein particles are elevated: VLDL and LDL or VLDL and increased numbers of cholesterol-depleted LDL particles can be recognized.

4.17 Anabolic Steroids

Hypercholesterolemia can occur in patients using anabolic steroids, reflecting the presence of an increased number of LDL particles, although reports differ as to whether this is, in fact, a significant side effect of these agents.

Pathophysiology of High LDL
The primary mechanism for hypercholesterolemia in patients using anabolic steroids is accumulation of LDL due to a reduction in the number of cell surface receptors for these particles, resulting in decreased catabolism of LDL.

Clinical Diagnosis
No diagnostic stigmata of high LDL are present on physical examination.

Treatment
Individuals who use anabolic steroids and have high LDL should stop anabolic steroids. High LDL should be treated aggressively due to a significantly increased risk of premature CAD. So, the first step is to stop anabolic steroids. Decreased dietary intake of saturated fat and simple carbohydrates, aerobic exercise, and weight loss can all have beneficial effects on the lipid profile. Patients with diabetes should be aggressively treated to maintain good glucose control. Statins should be the primary pharmacological agent to lower apoB (< 0.75 g/l).

5. ApoB in Cardiovascular Risk Prediction

Which marker of the apoB lipoproteins should we use to estimate cardiovascular risk: LDL-C, non-HDL-C or apoB?

- The LDL-associated risk of vascular disease is primarily due to the number of LDL particles and not to the mass of cholesterol within them. Therefore, LDL-C, the mass of cholesterol within all the LDL particles, is not an accurate marker of LDLassociated risk.
- ApoB measures the number of VLDL, IDL and LDL particles; non-HDL-C (total cholesterol - HDL-C) measures the total mass of cholesterol within the VLDL, IDL and LDL particles.
- Both apoB and non-HDL-C can be measured in non-fasting blood samples.
- Discordance analysis consistently demonstrates that apoB is a more accurate marker of cardiovascular risk than either LDL-C or non-HDL-C.

5.1 Introduction

In 2001, Adult Treatment Panel II (ATPII) added non-HDL-C as an alternative to LDL-C to estimate risk and to guide therapy in hypertriglyceridemic patients.[193] In 2012 and 2013, first the European lipid guidelines[194] and then the Canadian Guidelines[195] confirmed LDL-C as the prime measure for clinical care but stated that non-HDL-C or apoB could be alternative measures to drive clinical decisions. In 2013, the ACC/AHA guidelines stated therapy should be based on regimens, not lipid targets, whereas in 2014, the Joint British Societies Guidelines (JBS3)[196] and the National Lipid Association[197] selected non-HDL-C as the preferred target of therapy.

That so many different groups have made so many different choices based essentially on the same evidence demonstrates that the outcome of a guideline depends in part on the evidence, but also on the interpretations of the evidence by those who write the guidelines. This means that the Guideline process – the framing of recommendations from evidence – is not replicable. Replicability is a defining characteristic of science. If Guideline recommendations are not replicable, they should not be accepted automatically and without question.

We will begin by defining the markers and what they measure. We will then summarize the results of the generations of epidemiological studies that assessed their relative values as markers of atherogenic risk. The literature is vast and uneven with evidence in favor of all possible positions. We will try to explain why.

5.2 Defining the Markers

5.2.1 LDL-C

As discussed in Chapter 1, LDL-C is the mass of cholesterol within all the LDL particles. Since the mass of cholesterol within an LDL particle can vary substantially (*Figure 1.10 and Figure 5.1*), LDL-C is not a reliable measure of LDL particle number. Thus, when cholesterol-enriched LDL particles are present, the risk predicted by LDL-C will be greater than the risk predicted by the number of LDL particles and, conversely, when cholesterol-depleted LDL particles are present, LDL-C will underestimate the risk predicted by LDL particle number. Only when the mass of cholesterol is average will the risk predicted by LDL-C be equivalent to the risk predicted by LDL particle number. To summarize, when the mass of cholesterol per apoB particle is more or less than average, LDL-C and apoB or LDL particle number are discordant and will make different predictions of risk. By contrast, when the mass of cholesterol per particle is average, the cholesterol and particle markers are concordant and will make similar predictions of risk. Discordance analysis allows the markers to be compared when their predictions are different and the differences will not be diluted by all the instances in which they would be the same.[198] We will use discordance analysis later to test these contrasting predictions whether LDL-C, non-HDL-C or apoB is the best marker of cardiovascular risk.

The measurement of LDL-C has major limitations, which have not received the attention the issue deserves. If LDL-C is calculated by the Friedewald formula, as it is in the majority of laboratories, a fasting blood sample is necessary and the measurement is, unfortunately, as evaluated by the American Association Clinical Chemistry, often not acceptably precise.[199] Not only is the measurement of LDL-C imprecise, it is also not standardized,[199] which means the results from one laboratory will not necessarily be the same as the results from another, which means that tracking and interpreting the results of therapy or even of spontaneous changes over time will be difficult, if not impossible. Importantly, these errors are random and random errors

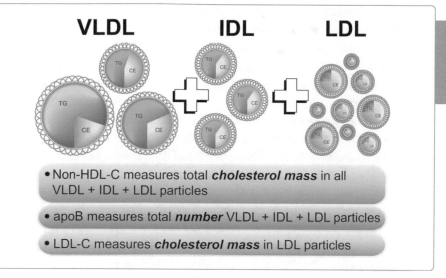

FIGURE 5.1

- Non-HDL-C measures total *cholesterol mass* in all VLDL + IDL + LDL particles

- apoB measures total *number* VLDL + IDL + LDL particles

- LDL-C measures *cholesterol mass* in LDL particles

due to imprecision of measurement cancel out in large surveys. Thus, the limitations that make LDL-C so poor a clinical tool for individual patients do not matter for the large studies that led guideline groups to recommend LDL-C as the standard of care.

On the other hand, if LDL-C is directly measured, as recommended by some guideline groups, there are multiple disadvantages[199]: 1) additional cost is added; 2) these methods are not standardized; 3) they are not validated in dyslipidemic serum; and 4) there is no epidemiological evidence that directly measured LDL-C is a more accurate measure of cardiovascular risk than the conventionally calculated LDL-C. Indeed the limited evidence available suggested the opposite to be the case.[200]

5.2.2 Non-HDL-C

Non-HDL-C is the arithmetic sum of the cholesterol in VLDL, IDL and LDL particles and, therefore, apoB and non-HDL-C seem like mirror images of each other with apoB measuring all the atherogenic particles and non-HDL-C measuring all the atherogenic cholesterol (Figure 5.1). No wonder so many argue that non-HDL-C is an acceptable surrogate for apoB and, given that no extra charge is required to calculate non-HDL-C, they conclude that non-HDL-C is superior to apoB. Furthermore, fasting samples are not required for non-HDL-C measurements and so apoB has no advantage on that front either.

Given that non-HDL-C includes the cholesterol in VLDL particles and given the high prevalence of hypertriglyceridemia in patients with vascular disease, it is not surprising that many experts attribute the increased cardiovascular risk in hypertriglyceridemic patients to so-called remnant particles within the VLDL density range. Unfortunately, the evidence that triglycerides increase risk remains incomplete. To be sure, recent Mendelian randomization studies suggest they do.[201-203] However, we are not sure confounding with LDL particle number has been ruled out in these analyses. There is certainly no linear relation between plasma triglyceride levels and risk, not surprising, since the highest levels are associated with increases in chylomicron number not VLDL particle number. Moreover – and this is a fundamental limitation – no evidence has yet been presented from any of the fibrate or niacin or even the statin clinical trials that any clinical benefit follows lowering of triglycerides or VLDL-C.

Finally, apoB48 and apoB100 abnormal remnant lipoprotein particles only accumulate in large numbers in patients with remnant lipoprotein disorder, when they can equal or exceed the normal VLDL particle number. In all other subjects the number of atherogenic remnant particles is indeed very low. Let us do an easy calculation: The normal fasting concentration of apoB48 is approximately 0.5 mg/ml and doubles in the peak postprandial period. The normal concentration of VLDL particles is 10 mg/dl, a value that also rises postprandially. Thus, normally, there are 10 to 20 times more VLDL particles than remnant particles. Remnant particles are atherogenic but the risk attributable to remnants must relate to their number and, if the number is not markedly increased, the risk attributable to remnants should not be markedly increased. Indeed, in healthy subjects, there are never very many atherogenic remnant particles. Only in remnant lipoprotein disorder is the concentration of abnormal VLDL and chylomicron remnants 40-50 mg/dl and therefore there are 20 to 40 times more in those with remnant lipoprotein disorder than in other subjects.[204] It is not surprising these patients have such an increased atherogenic risk.

Why Does VLDL-C not Explain Why non-HDL-C is a Better Marker of Cardiovascular Risk than LDL-C?

Based on our meta-analysis,[205] as well as other evidence, we have concluded that non-HDL-C is a more accurate marker of cardiovascular risk than LDL-C. However, not all studies, the Emerging Risk Factor Collaboration (ERFC)[206,207] for example, support this view. Those who conclude that non-HDL-C is superior to LDL-C assume this is due to the fact that non-HDL-C includes the cholesterol in VLDL and this increases the atherogenic risk. We will now try to demonstrate why this argument, which seems so common sense as to be inarguable, is more complex and less persuasive than it seems.

To begin with, since non-HDL-C is the simple sum of VLDL-C and LDL-C, this argument presumes the cholesterol in VLDL is as atherogenic as the cholesterol in LDL. But there is no direct evidence this is the case and given that LDL particles are so much smaller than VLDL particles and that there are so many more of them – 9 times more generally – the proposition the cholesterol in the much smaller number of the much larger VLDL particles is as dangerous, mmol for mmol, as the cholesterol in the much larger number of much smaller LDL particles seems, on the surface of it, unlikely. Nevertheless, let us examine in more detail the argument that the cholesterol in VLDL explains why non-HDL-C is a better marker of cardiovascular risk than LDL-C. The conventional method to express the risk attributable to any marker is the hazard ratio (HR), which is the increase in risk for one standard deviation increase in that marker. If non-HDL-C is a more accurate marker of cardiovascular risk than LDL-C, the HR for non-HDL-C must be greater than the HR for LDL-C. If the cholesterol in VLDL is the reason for this difference, then the HR of VLDL-C must be greater than the HR of LDL-C. Indeed, the HR VLDL-C must be greater than the HR of non-HDL-C.

The conclusion that follows from this elementary mathematics is that the cholesterol in VLDL poses a greater risk than the cholesterol in LDL. This seems highly improbable since LDL particles are so much smaller than VLDL particles and there are nine times more LDL particles than VLDL particles. Moreover, if this were actually true, based on the same elementary mathematics, it is easy to show that as VLDL-C gets less and less, it gets more and more dangerous.[208] If the answer, which seems so obvious, is wrong, what is the right answer?

Non-HDL-C is a Better Marker of Cardiovascular Risk than LDL-C Because it is an Indirect Way of Measuring LDL Particle Number

Let us start with what happens when VLDL particles interact with LDL particles in the presence of cholesterol ester transfer protein (CETP) as illustrated in Figure 1.12

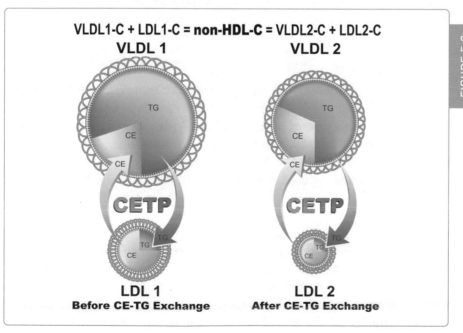

VLDL1-C + LDL1-C = **non-HDL-C** = VLDL2-C + LDL2-C

VLDL 1   VLDL 2

LDL 1   LDL 2
Before CE-TG Exchange   **After CE-TG Exchange**

FIGURE 5.2

and Figure 5.2. CETP promotes the exchange of the core lipids – cholesterol esters and triglyceride – between VLDL and LDL with the result that cholesterol ester is transferred in net amounts from LDL to VLDL and triglyceride from VLDL to LDL. The transfer of the cholesterol ester from LDL to VLDL produces the cholesterol-depleted LDL particle and because the LDL particle is cholesterol depleted, LDL-C underestimates the number of LDL particles. On the other hand, the cholesterol that has been removed from LDL particles reappears within the VLDL particles, thus increasing the VLDL-C. Accordingly as illustrated in Figure 5.2, non-HDL-C before the transfer is the same, at least hypo-thetically, as the non-HDL-C after the transfer because the lower LDL-C after transfer is balanced by the higher VLDL-C after transfer. This means that non-HDL-C restores the relation between LDL-C and LDL particle number and that the increase in non-HDL-C due to the transfer of cholesterol ester from LDL to VLDL restores the total relation of cholesterol within the apoB particles to the number of LDL particles.

Once this is grasped, it is not surprising that the correlation between non-HDL-C and apoB is significantly greater than the correlation between LDL-C and apoB and even more tellingly, the correlation between non-HDL-C and LDL particle number is greater than the correlation between LDL-C and LDL particle number. The bottom line, therefore, is that the reason that non-HDL-C is a more accurate marker of risk than LDL-C is that non-HDL-C is, in fact, just a backwards and indirect way of measuring LDL particle number. Accordingly, the superiority of non-HDL-C over LDL-C in no way supports the argument that lowering VLDL-C will produce clinical benefit. This may be so, but it has yet to be shown, and it needs to be shown before acting as if it were true.

5.2.3 ApoB

Total plasma apoB includes all the apoB particles, such as the VLDL and IDL particles and the Lp(a) particles as well as the LDL particles (see Figure 5.1). With few excep-tions, there are 9 times more LDL than VLDL apoB particles and the two exceptions can be recognized. These are remnant lipoprotein disorder and when plasma tri-glycerides are > 3.0 mmol/l.[88,209] Thus, in the vast majority of individuals, plasma apoB is determined by LDL apoB. LDL apoB can be measured directly but this requires isolation of the LDL from plasma by ultracentrifugation and therefore is not clinically practical. However, LDL apoB can be calculated from total cholesterol, HDL-C and triglyceride so long as plasma triglycerides are <3.0 mmol/l.[204] Given there is no evidence we are aware of that total apoB is a significantly stronger predictor of risk than LDL apoB, therefore, we believe that plasma apoB is acting as a surrogate for LDL apoB.

Fasting samples are not required to measure apoB because there are so few apo-B48 particles. The measurement of apoB is standardized and the American Association of Clinical Chemistry has determined that apoB can be measured more accurately in routine clinical laboratories than either LDL-C or non-HDL-C.[210] The perception of difficulties in the measurement of apoB relates to research studies, which used in-house, non-standardized methods or analyzed samples that had been preserved for very extended periods of time. Importantly, the cost of measuring apoB is low – less than 3 Euros or 5 Canadian or American dollars.

5.3 Summarizing the Evidence as to Whether LDL-C, non-HDL-C or ApoB is the Best Marker of Cardiovascular Risk

Lack of evidence is not the challenge. The challenge is the quality of much of the evidence. The quality of a study is based on its design, its methods, the precision with which it was executed, and the intelligence and scrupulousness with which it was interpreted. Epidemiological studies are powerful tools, but like any tool they have their limitations. The largest or even the most analytically sophisticated studies are not always the best studies because the data on which they are based may not be of high quality. If apoB or LDL-C, for example, were not measured accurately, the most sophisticated mathematical prestidigitations to analyze the data could not overcome the burden of inaccurate data and yield a valid answer. Moreover, with the exception of discordance analysis, none of the statistical analytical methods that have been used were designed to separate variables that closely correlate with each other as LDL-C, non-HDL-C and apoB so obviously do.

In this case, one marker is not absolutely right and the other two absolutely wrong. They are closely related physiologically; therefore they will be closely related epidemiologically. Nevertheless, while they are close, they are not the same. They are flashlights, pointed into the same darkness. But they differ in brightness and direction and therefore in just how much they make the shadows recede. Surely, we should include the brightest in our bag of diagnostic tools and it would be even better if we could join their illuminative powers. Thus our real objective is to demonstrate how by integrating the information – by considering LDL C, non-HDL C and apoB simultaneously in the individual and by using them as complimentary and not competitive measures – confusion and dispute dissipate. That, in fact, is the point of the apoB algorithm in which integrating total cholesterol, triglycerides and apoB makes diagnosis possible. Nevertheless, because it is an important issue, we will now summarize the evidence as to which marker is the best marker of cardiovascular risk.

5.3.1 Era 1 – Case-Control Studies

Case-control studies make up the first group of studies and, in general, these showed that apoB was superior to LDL-C and, in a smaller number, that non-HDL-C was superior to LDL-C.[210a] ApoB in these studies was usually measured by in-house immuno-assays, although in at least one instance, a chemical assay was used. These assays varied in quality and were not standardized. Nevertheless, during this period, the physico-chemical explanation for the observed superiority of apoB was reliably worked out. That is, LDL particles were shown to differ in the mass of cholesterol they contain and the principal mechanisms responsible were gradually elucidated. Until this was done, the charge was repeatedly made that any differences that were observed were, at best, due to differences in immunochemical reactivity. However, at this point in time, no one can challenge the mass of evidence that apoB particles do differ in size and composition.

5.3.2 Era 2 – Prospective Observational Studies

Prospective observational studies make up the second group of studies. The Quebec Cardiovascular Study was the first to show apoB was superior to LDL-C[211,212] and the AMORIS study was the largest.[213] Not all of these studies favored apoB. Differences in design complicated the issue. Some, such as ARIC, compared apoB with the sum of multiple lipid parameters including HDL-C.[214] Moreover, the quality of the methods to measure apoB also varied substantially. In ARIC, two methods were used, each with a coefficient of variation of > 15%, a value so large as to invalidate the results.

Only two attempts were made to integrate individual studies. The first was a conventional meta-analysis of all the studies that had reported results on LDL-C, non-HDL-C and apoB.[205] This study demonstrated that non-HDL-C was superior to LDL-C and apoB was superior to non-HDL-C. Moreover, when projected to the American population, the differences were large enough to matter. If ATPIII criteria were applied to select those who were to be treated and a 40% reduction in each marker were to be achieved, a reduction that is realistic in this day and age, applying quantitative projective analysis, we could show that using apoB would prevent 500,000 more cardiovascular events over 10 years than using LDL-C and that using apoB would prevent an additional 200,000 more events than using non-HDL-C.

If our meta-analysis yielded a positive picture for apoB, the participant level analysis by the Emerging Risk Factors Collaboration (ERFC) produced just the opposite result.[206,207] Not only were LDL-C, non-HDL-C and apoB equal in predictive power for cardiovascular events, none of these was superior to total cholesterol. Since total cholesterol can be measured more accurately and more cheaply than any of the other markers, the logical conclusion from ERFC is that total cholesterol should be the prime marker of cardiovascular risk. On the other hand, if ERFC is right, not only is our meta-analysis wrong but so are all the studies which showed that total cholesterol, LDL-C, non-HDL-C, were not equivalent markers to identify cardiovascular risk.

We think it is the conclusions from ERFC that are wrong, not the entire body of work that preceded and followed it. ERFC is a participant level analysis, which means that individual data from different studies are combined. Not all the data from any study will necessarily be included because ERFC inclusion criteria must be met. Therefore, the sample is *de novo*, defined by criteria that were not necessarily the same as those of the original study. Indeed, so many subjects may be eliminated that the study is no longer representative of the group that it purports to study. Moreover, unlike meta-analysis, there is no obligation to collect all the relevant data. Only the data from the investigators who participate are included in a participant level analysis. Selectivity of input – with all the risks involved – is built into the method. Even more important in this case is that different methods to measure lipids and apoB are merged in the same database. Many different methods were used to measure apoB. Most were not standardized and many were not accurate. Many samples were analyzed after prolonged periods, up to 20 years, in a freezer without evidence that the samples were safely preserved. Finally, many of the studies included in ERFC never published their methods or results and therefore data of the lower quality becomes equal to data of the higher quality.

5.3.3 Era 3 – Discordance Analysis: The Challenge of Separating Closely Correlated Variables

The issue we are concerned with – comparing the predictive accuracy of apoB to the cholesterol indices – poses a problem that none of the conventional analytical methods were designed to deal with. In this instance, we clinicians cannot simply turn the problem over to the statisticians. We must add the dimensions of knowledge that are natural to us to aid them to improve their analytical analysis. That is what we will try to do in this next section.

Correlation versus Concordance

Correlation is the rate of change of one variable versus the rate of change of another. High correlation has been taken as evidence two variables provide the same information. But high correlation is not adequate to establish whether two diagnostic measures are clinical equivalents. Their concordance must also be taken into account (Figure 5.3). Concordance is the range of values of one variable for any specific value of another. That is, if one variable is known, the dispersion of likely values for the other represents their concordance. Two measures may be highly correlated and also highly concordant as illustrated in Figure 5.3 – left panel. Therefore, in this example, one variable is clinically equivalent to the other: that is, from the value of one, you are very likely to know the value of the other. However, not all variables that are highly correlated are also highly concordant. This is illustrated in Figure 5.3 – right panel in which it is obvious that any particular value of one variable is associated with a wide range of values for the other. In this circumstance, the two variables are not clinically equivalent because, in the in-

FIGURE 5.3

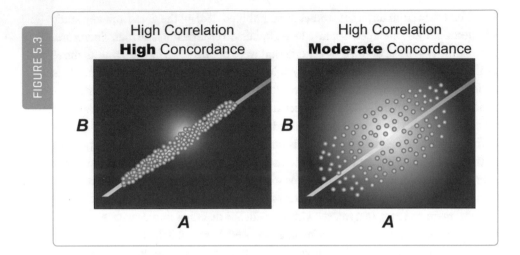

dividual, one cannot be substituted for the other. That is, they are highly correlated but they are discordant.

Discordance Analysis

LDL-C and apoB are highly correlated because all apoB particles contain substantial amounts of cholesterol. Non-HDL-C and apoB are even more highly correlated (0.85 to 0.90), so highly correlated that on this basis alone, groups such as ATPIII[215] and the JBS3 [196] have decided they are clinically equivalent. The first demonstration that this conclusion may be wrong came from a discordance analysis of LDL-C versus apoB and non-HDL-C versus apoB in the Quebec Cardiovascular Study.[216] For this study, concordance was defined as both values being within the same quintile. At the extremes, there was little discordance whereas over most of the distribution of values, there is substantial discordance – that is, values for one marker may be substantially different from the other.

Discordance analysis compares the accuracy of markers when they disagree and excludes those that agree. Conventional methods include both, therefore diluting the power to identify significant differences in predictive accuracy. The Framingham Heart Study was the first to formally apply this approach in the comparison of LDL particle number and LDL-C.[217]

The results were straightforward and striking. Four Kaplan-Meir survival curves are illustrated in Figure 5.4. Two groups are concordant for LDL-C and LDL particle number (LDL-P) while two groups are discordant. The two concordant groups – high LDL-C and LDL-P and low LDL-C and low LDL-P – demonstrate the expected differences in survival. Survival is reduced with a high LDL-C and a high LDL-P and enhanced with a low LDL-C and a low LDL-P. The key comparisons are the outcomes in the

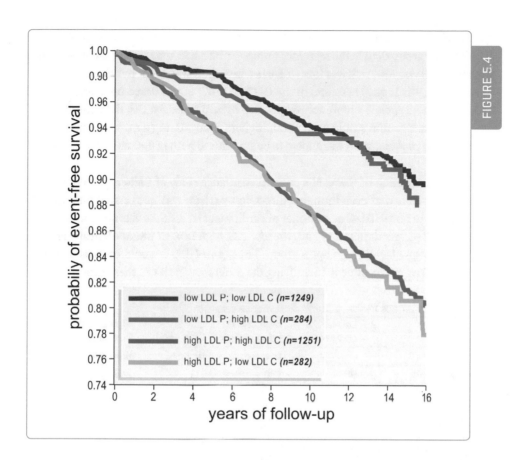

FIGURE 5.4

discordant groups. When LDL-C is high but LDL-P is low, that is, when cholesterol-enriched LDL particles are present, survival corresponds almost exactly to survival in the group with the low LDL-C and low LDL-P. That is, survival is good in both groups and LDL-P, not LDL-C, correctly identified the outcome. By contrast, when LDL-C is low but LDL-P is high – that is, when increased numbers of cholesterol-depleted LDL particles are present – survival is reduced in the discordant group and the outcome corresponds almost exactly to survival in the group with high LDL-C and high LDL-P. The conclusion could not be clearer – outcome is determined by LDL-P, not by LDL-C. So far as LDL particles are concerned, the critical variable is particle number, not particle composition. This result was also reproduced in the MESA study.[218] As well, in the Women's Heart Study, using discordance analysis, Mora and Ridker demonstrated that LDL-P, non-HDL-C and apoB were each superior to LDL-C.[219]

However, most attention has focused on whether apoB is superior to non-HDL-C as a marker of cardiovascular risk. A discordance analysis of apoB versus non-HDL-C in the INTERHEART study revealed that cardiovascular risk was less in the cholesterol-enriched discordant group than in the reference group and greater in the cholesterol-depleted group than in the reference group.[220,221] That is, when non-HDL-C was high and apoB was low, risk was low whereas when apoB was high, but non-HDL-C was low, risk was high. Therefore, in the INTERHEART study, based on a head-to-head comparison, apoB is a more accurate marker of cardiovascular risk than non-HDL-C.

The same findings hold in the Framingham Study. Using a novel method of discordance analysis, apoB was shown to be superior to both LDL-C and non-HDL-C.[221a]

Finally, inspection of the results of the discordance study of Ridker and Mora[219] also makes it clear that even though a direct comparison was not carried out, apoB is superior to non-HDL-C as a marker of cardiovascular risk. As is evident in Table 5.1, non-HDL-C was the same in both the low-risk high LDL-C/ low apoB group and the high-risk low LDL-C/high apoB group. Thus, non-HDL-C would be inaccurate just as LDL-C was inaccurate in identifying the difference in risk in these groups.

Table 5.1 Womens health study:[219] discordance analysis

	Low LDL-C Low apoB	High LDL-C Low apoB	Low LDL-C High apoB	High LDL-C High apoB
	Low risk	Low risk	High risk	High risk
LDL-C mg/dl	98	130	111	148
LDL-C mmol/l	2,54	3,37	2,87	3,84
Non-HDL-C mg/dl	125	157	152	185
Non-HDL-C mmol/l	3,25	4,08	3,95	4,81
apoB mg/dl	81	93	112	124
apoB g/l	0,81	0,93	1,12	1,24
TG mg/dl	93	94	182	149
TG mmol/l	1,05	1,06	2,06	1,68

To conclude there are multiple studies – six to date – based on discordance analysis, all of which show measures of apoB particle number are superior to measures of cholesterol mass – both non-HDL-C and LDL-C – to estimate cardiovascular risk. This methodology is more robust to test closely correlated variables than the conventional approaches and therefore the results, we suggest, are compelling.

6. ApoB Lipoprotein Particles: the preferred Treatment Target in Primary and Secondary Prevention

- Statin therapy lowers plasma apoB particle number, most of which are LDL apoB particles, and this reduction is why the rates of cardiovascular events are substantially reduced by statin therapy.
- Inaccurate measurement of this effect undercuts accurate therapy. That is why neither LDL-C nor non-HDL-C should be the preferred treatment targets to lower cardiovascular risk with LDL-lowering therapy.
- We recommend the use of apoB as the preferred target of therapy because:
  1. apoB can be measured more accurately and precisely than either non-HDL-C or LDL-C;
  2. apoB, like non-HDL-C, does not require fasting;
  3. decreases in apoB are more closely tied to benefit than decreases in LDL-C or non-HDL-C;
  4. apoB is a more accurate marker than either LDL-C or non-HDL-C of inadequate or incomplete LDL-lowering therapy.

We recommend a two-step target approach:
  1. Ensure apoB is lowered to < 0.75 g/l (~26th) percentile of the population);
  2. In those at very high risk and who are good candidates for intensive therapy, apoB should be lowered to < 0.65 g/l (~13th) percentile of the population).

The two-step apoB approach ensures that all patients who warrant therapy receive adequate therapy and that those in whom risk is particularly high are considered for optimal LDL-lowering therapy.

6.1 Introduction

LDL is the major proatherogenic apoB lipoprotein particle and statin therapy to lower LDL particle number in plasma substantially lowers the rates of cardiovascular events. Accordingly, every Guideline advocates statin therapy as fundamental to cardiovascular care. Nevertheless, notwithstanding that every guideline states they are evidence-based and all cite the same evidence, they do not agree on how to do it: that is, how much statin to give and what marker, if any, to assess the adequacy of therapy. The most recent European[222] and Canadian guidelines[195] recommend a target-based approach with LDL-C as the primary target and non-HDL-C and apoB as alternate targets. However, the Europeans have three targets and three intensities of therapy depending on the perceived level of risk whereas the Canadians have only one target level for each of the three markers and, therefore, only one intensity of therapy. On the other hand, the Joint British Societies[196] and the National Lipid Association[197] favor non-HDL-C as the best marker to judge the adequacy of LDL-lowering therapy (Table 6.1). Thus, as is obvious in Table 6.1, there is considerable variation in the targets for LDL-C, non-HDL-C and apoB amongst the different guidelines. Indeed for high-risk patients, the targets for LDL-C expressed in population percentiles differ between the 12th to 33rd percentile whereas apoB percentile targets vary between the 35th and 67th percentile.

All these approaches have been criticized by the ACC/AHA guidelines[223] on the grounds that the major statin trials actually tested regimens, not targets, and therefore all patients should receive the same standard dose of statin without adjustment based on any measure of LDL. This No Target/Regimen Only approach is diametrically opposed to the target strategies but is also evidence-based, actually, paradoxically, on the same evidence on which the target strategies are based. Because therapy is one of the most important issues we deal with, we must try to understand the relative strengths and weaknesses of these two different treatment strategies for LDL lowering. Based on this analysis, we will present the option we prefer – the apoB two-step approach, which we believe is the most clinically and physiologically appropriate approach given all the evidence and the limitations in the evidence.

Table 6.1 Targets for LDL-C, non-HDL-C and apoB in different international guidelines, expressed in units and in population percentiles.

Guideline	LDL-C mmol/l			Non-HDL-C			apoB	
	Concentration mmol/l mg/dl		NHANES population percentile	Concentration mmol/l mg/dl		NHANES population percentile	Concentration g/l	NHANES population percentile
National Lipid Association[197]								
High risk	< 2,6	< 100	33%	< 3,4	< 130	42%		
Very high risk	< 1,8	< 70	8%	< 2,6	< 100	16%		
ACC/AHA[223]								
High risk	< 2,6	< 100	33%	< 3,4	< 130	42%	< 0,9	51%
Very high risk	< 1,8	< 70	8%	< 2,6	< 100	16%	< 0,8	35%
EAS/ESC[194]								
High risk	< 2,6	< 100	33%	< 3,4	< 130	42%	< 1,0	67%
Very high risk	< 1,8	< 70	8%	< 2,6	< 100	16%	< 0,8	35%
Joint British Society 3[196]								
High risk and Very high risk	< 2,0	< 77	12%	< 3,0	< 115	27%		
Canadian Cardiovascular Society[195]								
High risk and very high risk	< 2,0	< 77	12%	< 2,6	< 100	16%	< 0,8	35%
EAS-HTG treatment target[197a]								
High risk							< 0,8	35%
Very high risk							< 0,7	19%

6.2 LDL Lowering Treatment Strategies

6.2.1 The No-Target/ Regimen Only-based Approach

The No-Target/Regimen Only approach states that the routine clinical regimen should be the regimen that was used in successful clinical trials. Clinical trials, the argument goes, tested regimens, not target levels and, therefore, it is regimens not targets that were validated by the clinical trials.[224] Moreover – the argument continues – lowering of LDL may not be the only mechanism of benefit from statins. Any of a number of other possible effects, such as reduction of inflammation, might be responsible for the so-called pleotropic clinical benefits of statins – that is, all the putative mechanisms other than LDL lowering that might produce clinical benefit by statins. Therefore, changes in LDL are not the only index of the therapeutic effects of statins from which it follows that changes in LDL should not govern the dose of statins. The premise for the argument is logical, but is the evidence for it complete and compelling?

The answer, unfortunately, is no. Amongst our reservations, the first is that six therapeutic trials – TNT,[225] GREACE,[226] AFCAPS/TexCAPS,[227] PROVE-IT TIMI,[225] MEGA[228] and Post-CABG[229] – did select doses in order to achieve a prespecified level of LDL. The number is not trivial and while the design of most as target trials may not be ideal and the evidence is incomplete, it is not non-existent.

Second, not all patients benefit equally, either clinically or in terms of LDL lowering, from the same dose of a statin. This distinction between individual and group benefit has been largely overlooked and that is unfortunate. The Cholesterol Treatment Trialists (CTT) meta-analysis of the cholesterol-lowering trials[230] concluded that the lowering of clinical events by a constant decrease in LDL-C is constant: that is, 1 mmol/l (38.5 mg/dl) reduction of LDL-C reduced clinical events by approximately 20%. Based on this finding, many have concluded that the relative benefit of statins is the same in all and the absolute benefit is determined by the absolute risk. In other words, all individuals are the same and the group response applies, therefore, to all.

But this conclusion does not follow from the CTT findings. If the relative benefit per mmol/l lowering of LDL-C is constant, then the absolute benefit possible depends on the baseline level of LDL-C because with each mmol/l reduction in LDL-C, risk is reduced by 20% from baseline. Thus, while the relative benefit per mmol/l lowering of LDL-C is constant, the absolute benefit depends on the baseline level of LDL-C.[231] Moreover – and this point also seems to have been overlooked – the absolute lowering of LDL-C by a statin depends not only on the dose and potency of the statin but also on the baseline level of LDL: the higher the baseline value, the greater the drop. It is the relative decrease in LDL produced by a statin that is constant not the absolute decrease.[232] Since, as we have just shown, benefit correlates with the absolute decrease in LDL, there will be greater benefit from the same dose and potency of a statin with higher baseline levels of LDL. Thus, it follows, logically and directly, from the CTT results[230] that not all patients benefit equally from statin therapy: those with higher levels achieve greater absolute benefit compared with those with lower levels (see Figure 7.4). Absolute benefit is meaningful clinically. Relative benefit can be misleading as the Guideline recommendations demonstrate. Unfortunately, this point is not widely appreciated.

Also not widely appreciated is that the change in LDL-C induced by a standard dose of a statin varies widely.[233] Rosuvastatin 20 mg daily, for example, reduces LDL-C, on average, by 40%, but in 10% of patients, the decrease in LDL-C is less than 20% whereas in 10%, the decrease in LDL-C is greater than 70%. For practical purposes, this means that adequate LDL lowering cannot be assumed to occur in all patients who are prescribed a standard dose of a statin. In our view, this is a fatal objection to the No Target/Regimen Only Strategy, given that the CTT meta-analysis demonstrates convincingly that, over the range of lowering of LDL achieved with statins, there is a direct relationship between benefit and the decrease achieved.[230] Without measuring levels of LDL, how can either the patient or the physician be sure the response is adequate? Without measuring the levels of LDL, how can the physician be sure the patient is even taking the statin?

ACC/AHA[223] dealt with this challenge by creating a protocol to determine whether the response to statin therapy was adequate. An adequate response was defined as at least a 50% decrease from the baseline level, failing which the statin dose or potency could be increased or ezetimibe might be added. Defining an adequate response to statin is in practical terms indistinguishable from defining a target and therefore much of the debate about the ACC/AHA guidelines seems moot.

Moreover, given the results of the IMPROVE-IT trial,[234] which demonstrated a modest – 5.7% – but real decrease in clinical events with lowering of LDL-C from to 1.81 mmol/l (70 mg/dl) to 1.37 mmol/l (53 mg/dl), the argument that benefit from LDL lowering is related to anything else but LDL lowering would seem to have little weight. On the other hand, the fact the actual event rate was only reduced from 34.7 to 32.7% would suggest there is a real limit to the absolute benefit achievable with LDL-lowering therapy. When LDL is already very low, the absolute potential gain from further lowering is, unfortunately, limited.

Third, the evidence base is too limited to allow an evidence-based choice of the intensity of statin therapy. Atorvastatin 80 mg daily may be superior to atorvastatin 10 mg daily as the limited available clinical trial evidence does suggest is the case. However, 10 mg atorvastatin will lower LDL-C by 75% of the total amount that 80 mg atorvastatin will.[235] Therefore, most of the benefit that can be achieved with statin therapy will be achieved with the initial doses. Nevertheless, somewhat more benefit could be clinically meaningful. But is atorvastatin 80 mg superior to atorvastatin 40 mg qd or to atorvastatin 20 mg qd? Perhaps, but there is no evidence to support any such conclusion because the doses have never been compared in a randomized clinical trial. Moreover, given the very small incremental lowering of LDL as statin doses are doubled (the rule of 6 – that is, each doubling of the dose of statin reduces LDL-C by 6%) and given the evidence that myalgia increases and compliance decreases as statin doses increase;[236-238] and given the evidence that the risk of statin-induced diabetes mellitus is dose-related[239] and that reduced adherence is associated with increased cardiovascular risk,[237,238,240] it is not reasonable to conclude that the highest dose is necessarily the best dose. And certainly, there is no RCT evidence this is the case.

Individually and together, in our view, these reservations sum to the conclusion that the evidence base for a No Target/Regimen Only-based strategy is not adequate.

6.2.2 The Target-Based Approach to LDL-Lowering Therapy

The target approach states LDL-lowering therapy should be adjusted to achieve a predetermined level of LDL. This has been the conventional model of care and LDL-C has been the conventional marker of LDL on which to base the target. We think this model of care can be modified with benefit, as we shall discuss below.

The target-based approach was developed by ATPIII[241] and was the choice of the most recent European,[222] Canadian,[195] British, as well as other recent Guidelines. However, the target-based strategy has important limitations. The first is that the majority of the statin trials were not designed to test targets of therapy but rather were, just as Hayward and Krumholtz[224] state, primarily designed to test two regimens – either a fixed dose of a statin against placebo or a fixed dose of a statin against a different fixed dose of the same or a different statin. That said, the weight of the evidence, which by this point is quite weighty, demonstrates beyond a reasonable doubt that lower levels of LDL post therapy are associated with greater overall benefit than higher levels of LDL post therapy. The caveat, however, as we have just reviewed, is that the absolute benefit from LDL lowering is related to the absolute level of LDL before therapy and the absolute lowering of LDL with therapy. It follows that the incremental absolute benefit with therapy becomes less as the levels of LDL become lower and lower.

Accordingly, benefit is not unlimited. Indeed, the relation of LDL to cardiovascular risk is curvilinear, not linear (Figure 6.1).

Thus risk increases exponentially as plasma levels of LDL increase and, conversely, risk decreases exponentially as plasma levels decrease. This means that as LDL levels become lower, LDL-attributable risk is lower. Evidence in support of this view comes from the results of Boekholdt et al. who calculated the hazard ratios for LDL-C, non-HDL-C and apoB in 8 statin clinical trials. These are shown in Table 6.2. Note that these

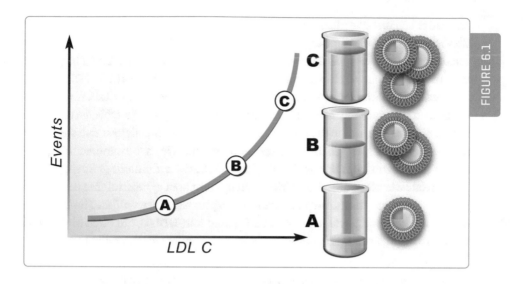

FIGURE 6.1

Table 6.2 Difference in risk prediction and risk reduction of an event by the three markers of plasma LDL in meta-analysis of prospective data versus on-treatment data in statin clinical trials.

Marker	Prospective Risk prediction Meta-analysis[242]	On-treatment Risk prediction Meta-analysis[244]	On-treatment Risk reduction Meta analysis[246]
LDL-C	1.25 [1.18-1.33]	1.13 [1.10-1.17]	20.1% [15.6%-24.3%]
Non-HDL-C	1.34 [1.24-1.44]	1.16 [1.12-1.19]	20.0% [15.2%-24.7%]
ApoB	1.43 [1.35 1.50]	1.14 [1.11-1.18]	24.4% [19.2%-29.2%]

were substantially lower than the hazard ratios obtained in a meta-analysis of prospective observational studies, an outcome which is consistent with lower LDL levels posing less risk.

This is also why the finding by Boekholdt et al.[242] that non-HDL-C, LDL-C and apoB predicted the risk of an event while on-treatment equally well is not surprising. Nor are the results of the Heart Protection Study (HPS)[243] which reported the same findings, surprising either. The LDL in these subjects was also low on average. Therefore the LDL-attributable risk was low and if LDL does not account for much of the event rate, it is unlikely there will be much difference in predictive accuracy amongst the markers. Nevertheless, this does not mean these markers are not of value to guide LDL-lowering therapy. Accordingly, we have examined the issue a different way by determining their relation to benefit rather than to risk.[244] Statins lower LDL-C and non-HDL-C more than they lower apoB[245] and the benefit from statin-induced LDL lowering is more closely related to changes in apoB than to changes in LDL-C or non-HDL-C.[244] That means that apoB is a better target of statin therapy than LDL-C or non-HDL-C (Table 6.2).

There is yet another point to consider. While the average levels of LDL were low in the treated groups of the recent major statin trials, not all patients achieved these low levels. Since risk relates to the level of LDL, those who are the highest risk should be the ones most likely to benefit from further treatment. We have examined this question in the 6 statin trials that achieved levels of LDL-C < 2.1 mmol/l (< 80 mg/dl).[246]

The relative levels of different markers can be compared by determining their levels in the population – that is, their relative levels expressed as percentiles. Thus, as Table 6.3 illustrates, apoB levels, relative to LDL-C and non-HDL-C, are often higher and therefore identify subjects in whom residual risk is more closely tied to LDL.[246]

Table 6.3 On-treatment LDL-C, non-HDL-c and apoB concentrations and NHANES population percentile.

	LDL-C			Non-HDL-C			apoB	
	Concen-tration		Population percentile	Concen-tration		Population percentile	Concen-tration	Population percentile
	mmol/l	mg/dl		mmol/l	mg/dl		g/l	
TNT 80 mg atorvastatin [1]	1,95	75	12%	2,62	101	14%	0,98	51%
IDEAL 80 mg atorvastatin [2]	2,08	80	15%	2,65	102	15%	0,84	29%
JUPITER 20 mg rosuvastatin [3]	1,43	55	3%	1,97	76	3%	0,66	9%
CARDS 10 mg atorvastatin [4]	1,87	72	11%	2,60	100	14%	0,80	25%
HPS 40 mg simvastatin [5]	2,08	80	15%				0,78	25%
PROVE-IT 80 mg atorvastatin [6]	1,61	62	5%				0,67	11%

Table reprinted from reference 246. 1. LaRosa JC, Grundy SM, Waters DD, et al. Intensive lipid lowering with atorvastatin in patients with stable coronary disease. N Engl J Med 2005; 352:1425–1435. Reference 225. 2. Pedersen TR, Faergeman O, Kastelein JJP, et al. High-dose atorvastatin vs usual-dose simvastatin for secondary prevention after myocardial infarction. The IDEAL Study: a randomized controlled trial. JAMA 2005; 294:2437-2445. 3. Ridker PM, Danielson E, Fonseca FA, et al. Rosuvastatin to prevent vascular events in men and women with elevated C-reactive protein. N Engl J Med 2008; 359:2195-2207. 4. Colhoun HM, Betteridge DJ, Durrington PN, et al. Primary prevention of cardiovascular disease with atorvastatin. Atorvastatin Diabetes Study (CARDS): multicentre randomised placebo controlled trial. Lancet 2004; 364:685-696. 5. Heart Protection Study Collaborative Group. MRC/BHF Heart Protection Study of cholesterol lowering with simvastatin in 20,536 high-risk individuals: a randomised placebo-controlled trial. Lancet 2002; 360:7-22. Reference 252. 6. Cannon CP, Braunwald E, McCabe CH, et al. Intensive versus moderate lipid lowering with statins after acute coronary syndromes. N Engl J Med 2004; 350:1495-1504.

6.2.3 The Two Step Target Approach

The Two Step approach is the strategy we favor and it is based on the reality that the limitations in the evidence and the complexities inherent in individual clinical care preclude a one-size-fits-all strategy. Moreover, our strategy is based on the use of apoB because apoB can be measured more accurately and precisely than either non-HDL-C or LDL-C;[199,210] because apoB, like non-HDL C, does not require fasting; because decreases in apoB are more closely tied to benefit than decreases in LDL-C or non-HDL-C; and because apoB is a much more accurate index than either LDL-C or non-HDL-C of inadequate or incomplete LDL-lowering therapy, as reviewed and discussed in Chapter 5. ApoB is also more accurately measured than either LDL-C or non-HDL-C and can be easily, accurately and inexpensively (approximately 5 Canadian dollars or 3 Euros) determined in any routine clinical chemistry laboratory.

Accordingly, Step 1 of our Two Step approach is to ensure apoB is lowered to < 0.75 g/l. A level of 0.75 g/l corresponds to the ~26th percentile of the population (Figure 6.2 and Appendix table). This value of apoB is equivalent to an LDL-C < 2.4 mmol/l and a

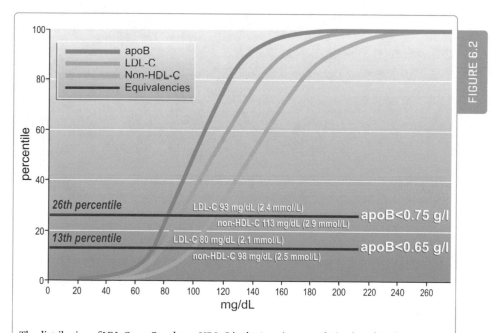

FIGURE 6.2

The distribution of LDL-C, apoB and non-HDL-C in the American population based on the NHANES survey (www.cdc.gov/nchs/nhanes). This allows the equivalent population percentiles for absolute concentrations of LDL-C, apoB and non-HDL-C to be determined and compared. The red lines indicate the apoB targets for high risk (< 0.75 g/l) and very high risk (< 0.65 g/l). In the Appendix all values of LDL-C, apoB and non-HDL-C by percentiles in the population are indicated.

non-HDL-C < 2.9 mmol/l – which for LDL-C corresponds to targets in high-risk patients in multiple guidelines (Table 6.1). Any level greater than this represents inadequate therapy. Therefore, we recommend that statin potency and dose should be adjusted to achieve a level < 0.75 g/l and that, if necessary, and clinically appropriate for that individual, a cholesterol inhibitor be added.

Step 2: An apoB of 0.75 g/l only represents the 26th percentile of the American population[247] and achieving this level does not mean that additional significant benefit from LDL lowering is not possible. That is why in those who are at very high risk and who are good candidates for intensive therapy, maximal LDL-lowering therapy is indicated to reach an apoB of 0.65 g/l – the 13th percentile of the American population and the level equivalent to the target levels of LDL-C (≤ 2.1 mmol/l and non-HDL-C (≤ 2.5 mmol/l) chosen by the Canadian Guideline Groups (Table 6.1).[195] Intensive therapy would mean full dose of a potent statin plus, if necessary, cholesterol absorption inhibitor. In the future, other agents, such as PCSK9 inhibitors, may also be available.

7. The Future of ApoB: Moving from the Risk Prediction Paradigm to the Causal Exposure Paradigm

The Risk Prediction Paradigm To Prevent Cardiovascular Events

- In the Risk Prediction Paradigm, medical preventive treatment is offered only after a predefined level of risk of a clinical event during the next decade is exceeded.

- Risk cannot be high until complex and extensive atherosclerotic lesions are present within the arterial wall and this is not common until the 60s in men and the 70s in women.

- Consequently, calculated risk will be low in individuals in early middle age with markedly abnormal blood pressure or LDL and preventive therapy triggered by risk will not be initiated in many until advanced disease is present. Accordingly the benefits of statin therapy may well be substantially diminished in many individuals.

- Moreover, the risk of a cardiovascular event can be predicted with acceptable precision in groups but not in individuals. This imprecision in the prediction of risk for an individual is not appreciated even though it represents a major flaw in the Risk Prediction Paradigm so far as individual care is concerned.

The Causal Exposure Paradigm To Prevent Cardiovascular Disease

- The atherogenic apoB lipoprotein particles, hypertension, and smoking all cause vascular disease. They are causes of, not risk factors for, cardiovascular disease.

- The damage these factors cause within the arterial wall is directly related to their magnitude and the length of time they are present.

- Since these causal factors injure the arterial wall over time, earlier intervention will arrest or sharply diminish the rate at which complex lesions develop within the arterial wall.

- In the absence of advanced lesions, the risk of a clinical event is virtually nil. Therefore, early intervention to treat hypertension and elevated apoB before advanced disease has developed should be a more effective strategy to prevent cardiovascular events than prevention that begins only after risk is high: that is, when advanced lesions are present.

7.1 Introduction

Words matter. The words we choose to represent our beliefs govern how we act. Accordingly, the objective of this final chapter is to argue that we should change our language so that we will change our actions. The Risk Prediction Paradigm presently governs prevention of vascular disease. However, we believe prevention would be much more successful if we moved to the Causal Exposure Paradigm, which is simpler, more direct, and calls for earlier therapeutic intervention than the Risk Prediction Paradigm.[231,248,249]

Although the algorithms to calculate risk differ, the levels of risk that prompt action differ, and the actions that are taken to lower risk differ, all the cholesterol guidelines [195-197,222,250,251] are governed by the Risk Prediction Paradigm, which dictates that medical preventive treatment is offered only after a predefined level of risk of a clinical event during the next decade is exceeded. To be sure, there are a number of exceptions, such as symptomatic vascular disease, extreme elevation of LDL-C or diabetes that automatically validate statin preventive therapy because risk is known to be high in all of these. Nevertheless, the primary consequence of this approach is to restrict statin preventive treatment to those who are asymptomatic but at calculated high risk of a clinical event over the next decade.

By contrast, we favor the Causal Exposure Paradigm,[231,249] which is based on identifying and treating the causal factors for vascular disease in individuals. The objective of the Causal Exposure Paradigm is to prevent the disease within the arteries that causes the clinical events because it is extensive anatomic atherosclerotic disease that eventually results in clinical events. The reality is that intramural disease is already advanced and extensive before obstructive focal lesions appear. At this point, only some of the anatomic complications of this advanced disease, which produce clinical events, can be prevented by statin therapy. Therefore, once predicted risk is elevated – that is, once the Risk Prediction Paradigm would call for prevention – extensive intramural disease is likely already present in many of those selected for preventive therapy and the gains of prevention, while real and substantial, will likely be limited and less than they would have been if therapy had started earlier (Figure 7.1).

FIGURE 7.1

Children	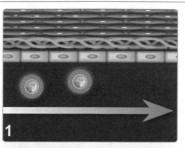	Picture 1-2-3-4 show a simplified scheme of the development of atherosclerotic lesions eventually resulting in clinical events.	
Young Adults Exposure to causal factors: LDL, blood pressure (BP), smoking	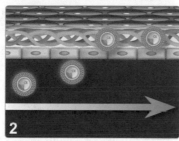	**Risk prediction paradigm** No risk of CV event < 10 years No treatment unless LDL or BP extremely high	**Causal Exposure Paradigm** High LDL & BP are causal factors of CVD Treatment of high LDL and elevated BP
Middle-aged Adults Asymptomatic lesions Age: < 60 yrs men < 70 yrs women	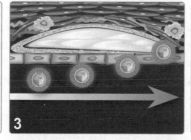	**Risk Prediction Paradigm** Increased lifetime CVD risk but low 10-yrs CVD risk: No primary prevention	**Causal Exposure Paradigm** High LDL & BP are causal factors of CVD Primary prevention indicated
Older Adults Advanced High Risk lesions Age: > 60 yrs men > 70 yrs women	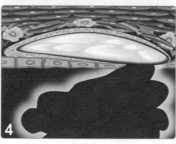	**Risk Prediction Paradigm** Increased risk of events in 10 years Primary Prevention indicated but only limited benefit possible because advanced complex lesions are present	**Causal Exposure Paradigm** High LDL & BP are causal factors of CVD Primary prevention indicated but only limited benefit possible because advanced complex lesions are present.

7.2 Strengths of the Risk Prediction Paradigm

The Risk Prediction Paradigm is based on the proposition that the costs and risks of pharmacological therapy are justified only in those who are likely in the immediate future to suffer a clinical event, a proposition that on the face of it seems inarguable. After all, it is clinical events that injure us and therefore it is clinical events we should want to prevent. In this approach, the impact of a limited number of factors – typically, total cholesterol, HDL-C, blood pressure (BP), treatment for elevated BP, smoking and diabetes – are integrated into a multiple regression algorithm that calculates the likelihood of a cardiovascular event over the next decade. Causes are transformed into calculated risk and decisions are based on calculated risk, not causes.

Moreover, based on the Heart Protection Study[252] and the meta-analyses of the CTT,[230] it has been widely accepted that the benefit of LDL lowering by statins is based on the level of risk, not on the level of LDL: the higher the risk, the greater the benefit; the lower the risk, the lower the benefit. In this scheme, the level of LDL is not relevant. Risk is all that matters. Furthermore, the AHA/ACC guidelines[250] have stated that the statin clinical trials were tests of regimens, not of targets, and therefore therapy should not be adjusted to achieve any particular level of any particular marker of LDL.

The primary strengths of the Risk Prediction Paradigm are: first, that it works in that the frequency of events over a decade in a group of individuals can be forecast with reasonable accuracy and, second, that it is so broadly accepted by clinical scientists that it has also been broadly accepted by societal decision-makers. Prevention based on risk appears to be a quantitative, inclusive, rational, judicious approach and so, it has become the dominant paradigm to prevent cardiovascular events, appropriately balancing the costs of the adverse clinical events as well as the costs of the therapies against the benefits. Nevertheless, however broadly and deeply accepted, we believe there are major limitations in this approach, which we will set out below.

7.3 Weaknesses of the Risk Prevention Paradigm

7.3.1 The Limitation of Basing the Decision to Treat on the Likelihood of a Clinical Event over the Next Decade

The phrase – Primary Prevention – suggests we are starting with a blank slate: an artery that is normal, pristine, inviolate and that appropriate therapy will prevent the initiation and maturation of atherosclerotic lesions, which invade and destroy the walls of a normal artery, converting it from a soft supple tube to a hard rigid one that may suddenly, without warning, severely narrow or occlude. Unfortunately, in the real world, such a hope of beginning therapy before disease is well seated within the arteries is too often false because advanced intramural atherosclerotic disease is a necessary prerequisite for clinical events. Simply put: a high calculated risk over the next decade reflects a high probability that significant intramural atherosclerotic disease is already present in a substantial number of individuals. Otherwise risk for the group could not be high. This tight and necessary connection between established disease and clinical risk seems so obvious that it should not need saying but a risk-based strategy that initiates prevention only after risk is elevated has ignored this reality.

We know that it takes time for advanced intramural disease to develop – almost always decades and decades, extremely rare disorders with extreme elevations of LDL such as homozygous familial hypercholesterolemia being the rare exceptions. Moreover, even though the natural history of atherosclerosis stretches out over decades, there is evidence that it progresses at different rates at different times. Thus, anatomic disease, at least in men, increases rapidly between 30 and 49, but appears to peak in terms of progression between 50 and 59, advancing steadily but less dramatically after that.[253] For much of this time, dilatation of the artery prevents encroachment of the lesions on the lumen and only after serious injury to the arterial wall has occurred do acute reductions in the lumen of an artery occur. Because significant disease takes so long to develop, cardiovascular events only become common, at least as expressed as a percent of the population, when men are 60 or more and women are 70 or more. Therefore, the risk of a clinical event over the next decade cannot be high until men and women have reached these ages at which point, based on age alone, most will be at high risk.

Not surprisingly, therefore, in the United States, based on the new AHA/ACC Guidelines, 90% of men and 50% of women over 60 will be at 'high risk' and eligible for therapy.[254] Indeed, a white male with no risk factors for CVD – that is a male who is a non-smoker, non-diabetic with a normal blood pressure and a normal non-HDL-C – will exceed the calculated 7.5% 10-year risk of a cardiovascular event at age 63 as will be the case for a 66-year-old African American man, a 70-year-old African American woman or a 71-year-old white woman. Age alone will take them over the treatment threshold. Age has this commanding power because the rate of events is relatively low before these ages but increases exponentially thereafter.

By the same token, age eliminates most of those who are under 60 as candidates for prevention, whether or not one of the cardinal causes of vascular disease – elevated LDL or blood pressure – is present. Consider a man with an LDL-C of 4.42 mmol/l (170 mg/dl), a level that is equivalent to the 94th percentile of the American population. At age 40, his 10-year risk is 2%, at age 50, 5%.[223] Only at age 60 would his calculated 10-year risk exceed the threshold at which prevention with statins would be definitely recommended.

But this delay may cost him dearly since sudden death or substantial and irreversible injury to his left ventricle may be the first clinical manifestations of cardiovascular disease. Early cardiovascular events are the most costly in personal and societal terms because the victim is cut down within the most productive phase of their life and those who depend on him or her and the society that profits from his or her contributions are also profound losers. Unfortunately also, such tragic events are by no means as rare as most believe. Yet because, at the moment, prevention is based on calculated risk, the majority of early victims would not have been eligible for therapy simply because they were too young.

However, an equally, if not even more important, argument against the Risk Prediction Paradigm – because it involves a so much larger number of people – is that the ultimate total benefit of prevention by LDL lowering will be diminished if preventive therapy is initiated only after advanced intramural atherosclerotic lesions have developed. The risk of a clinical event in the 40-year-old man with the markedly elevated LDL-C might well be only 2% over the next decade and only 5% over the decade to follow. But during all of these 20 years, his arterial tree is under continuous assault from the LDL particles, which will enter and be trapped within the wall and which will drive the development and maturation of complex advanced intramural disease. The disease, which develops during this time, is the reason that his risk rises at age 60. Delaying LDL-lowering therapy has allowed this to occur unchallenged.

The cost in terms of events that might have been avoided may be considerable since clinical events may result from statins from multiple pathophysiological mechanisms, only some of which are inhibited or interfered with by statins. Thus the endothelium can be eroded and platelets adhere and clump to the denuded surface.[255] This can produce a platelet-rich thrombus, which then detaches and embolizes downstream occluding a smaller vessel infarcting the muscle it supplies. A sequence such as this is a particularly common cause of sudden death and statins are unlikely to reduce the likelihood of this unhappy event. Alternatively, the fibrous cap can rupture, tearing the endothelium above it, exposing the thrombogenic lipid core directly to the blood, producing an acute occlusive thrombosis at the site. The likelihood of cap rupture is determined by multiple independent factors that affect its integrity: deposition of cholesterol in the core, the collagen production by smooth muscle cells, the activity of metalloproteinases from inflammatory cells, which can hydrolyze the collagen, systolic blood pressure and sympathetic stimulation of the heart, which alter mechanical stress and strain on the artery.[256,257] Hemorrhage in the subadventitial space from the neovascularization that has developed in response to the injury within the arterial wall is yet another possibility.[258] The hemorrhage can swell the thickness of the wall and reduce or occlude the lumen of the vessel.

Thus, there are multiple mechanisms of clinical events, each of which has a specific pathophysiology and therefore a specific set of inciting factors, and what finally happens depends on many intermediate steps. Statins are a potent therapy to reduce clinical events. But they are an imperfect therapy. Only a portion of the events recorded in the clinical trials are ever avoided, presumably because statins are effective against only some of the mechanisms that produce events. Thus, statins are likely to reduce the risk of plaque rupture because the deposition of cholesterol is reduced and the fibrous cap may consequently be strengthened but they are less likely to affect spontaneous intramural hemorrhage or endothelial denudation.

The bottom line is that once extensive intramural atherosclerotic disease is present, statins or any other form of LDL lowering will only be partially successful. This argues strongly that prevention should begin when we identify the causes of intravascular disease not when risk is high because disease will already be far advanced at this point. This is too often the fatal flaw in the Risk Prediction Paradigm.

7.3.2 Why is the Absolute Benefit of Statin Therapy Higher in Secondary Rather Than Primary Prevention?

The absolute benefit of statin therapy is significantly greater in secondary prevention than in primary prevention. But this is due to the fact that cardiovascular risk is more homogenous in individuals who have suffered a clinical event than in those who have not, and this homogeneity is not due to any intrinsic difference in the potency of statins in those who are truly at risk. Advanced atherosclerotic disease is an essential precondition for a clinical cardiovascular event. Therefore, all patients eligible for secondary prevention are at substantial risk of a clinical event because all have advanced anatomic atherosclerotic disease at the onset of the trial. In this sense, patients for secondary prevention are homogenous with regard to risk. Certainly, risk is not identical for all because there are multiple determinants of outcome in these patients; but all are at elevated risk.

By contrast, patients selected for primary prevention are severely heterogeneous with regard to risk. Conceptually, at least three subgroups can be distinguished.[231] A substantial subgroup would not have any lesions that were sufficiently advanced or unstable as to be capable of producing a clinical event within the limited time frame that a clinical trial lasts. Accordingly, this subgroup has effectively a zero risk of a cardiovascular event during the 5 years of follow-up. A second subgroup starts the 5-year period of the clinical trial with lesions that are more than minimal and, over the 5 years of the trial, these lesions advance with the result that complex, high-risk lesions appear during the subsequent 5-10 years, lesions that are capable of producing clinical events. These individuals do not contribute events during the limited 5-year time course of the clinical trial but may sustain events following the trial. Finally, individuals in the third subgroup have advanced but asymptomatic lesions at the onset of the 5-year period. These lesions have the same physical characteristics (inflamed, lipid-rich lesions that are vulnerable to fissuring or rupturing) as those in patients who have already suffered a clinical event and, therefore, the same likelihood of suffering an acute coronary syndrome.

With this background, let us perform a hypothetical RCT on the benefits of statin therapy in primary and secondary prevention.[231] Let the cardiovascular risk of a group of subjects with symptomatic cardiovascular disease be 20%. Based on the CTT meta-analysis,[230] 40 mg simvastatin will reduce their cardiovascular event rate from 20% to 16% with treatment for 5 years (Figure 7.2).[172] In a parallel primary prevention study, let us assume that 20% of the primary prevention group have sufficiently advanced anatomic disease that they could suffer a clinical cardiovascular event within the 5 years of the clinical trial. These subjects correspond to the third subgroup just discussed within the overall cohort of those who would receive primary prevention. Again, based on CTT, simvastatin should be just as effective in this subgroup as in those with secondary prevention. If so, 40 mg simvastatin will reduce the event rate in the total group from 4% to 3.2% (Figure 7.3).

FIGURE 7.2

Secondary Prevention
+ 40 mg Simvastatin

FIGURE 73

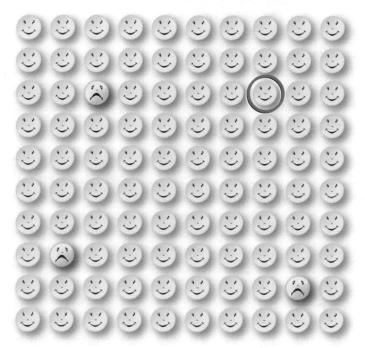

Primary Prevention
+ 40 mg Simvastatin

Thus, absolute benefit is much higher in secondary than primary prevention – 4% vs. 0.8% – just as the randomized clinical trials have demonstrated. However, for those individuals in both arms who could actually benefit, the relative gain is the same. Moreover, to whom in the primary prevention group does the average risk of 4% apply? The average arises from only 20% of the group: 80% are effectively at 0% risk while the other 20% are at 20% risk. Of course, we have simplified this though experiment because individual risk is not identical in any subgroup. But the core reasoning remains valid and the example illustrates that the observed differences in the real world appear to be the consequence of our not being able to select those who have already developed disease within the group eligible for primary prevention. Risk is calculated for groups and we presume that any particular individual within a group is at the same risk as any other individual within the group. While risk for all those with symptomatic vascular disease is obviously not identical, there is no substantial low-risk subgroup. For primary prevention, that is not the case. This is an important limitation of the Risk Prediction paradigm.

Moreover – and this benefit is not generally appreciated – statin therapy will benefit those individuals in primary prevention not only in subgroup 3, those with advanced disease, but will also benefit individuals in subgroup 2, those with minimal to moderate disease, by inhibiting the progression of atherosclerotic disease over the 5 years of a primary prevention trial. By inhibiting the progression of lesions and by increasing their stability, clinical benefit will not be realized during the clinical trial but in the future. The limited period of time of the clinical trial, therefore, limits our ability to measure the full clinical benefit of the statin regimen for primary prevention.

7.3.3 How Accurately Does the Risk Prediction Paradigm Predict Clinical Events for a Specific Individual?

Any prediction generated on the basis of individual data is assumed to be the risk for that specific individual. It is their personal risk. Certainly that is how we, as physicians, discuss the issue with a patient. Yet it is not so simple. If we tell an individual that he or she faces a 7.5% chance of a cardiovascular event over the next 10 years, does that mean that 7.5 times out of 100, he or she will suffer a cardiovascular event over the next 10 years? Obviously not, since he or she, like all of us, live only once, not 100 times.

But if the prediction is not literally meaningful – notwithstanding that is the form in which it was presented – is it even a valid scientific statement? No again, because at the end of 10 years, we will know whether a particular individual suffered an event or not, but we will not know whether the probability that we forecast was correct. Simply put, there is no way, looking backwards, to judge whether the prediction, looking forwards, was correct. This is unfortunate because scientific statements must be verifiable or they are not scientific statements. Guidelines cannot suspend this rule simply because it is convenient to do so – or at least they should not be able to do so.

The reply, of course, is always delivered authoritatively that this is the predicted risk of a group of individuals, each of whom is at the same calculated risk or within the same narrow range of calculated risks. This type of prediction can be directly validated and, if it is, the algorithm is said to be well calibrated and the result applies to the individual. But are the results of even a well-calibrated model transferable to the individuals from whom it was derived? Yes, but only if risk is homogenous within the individuals that make up the group. Unfortunately, this is usually not the case as the example of primary prevention presented above illustrates.

A second line of analysis – net reclassification – demonstrates directly the fundamental nature of the error. Thus, based on the results of coronary calcification, groups of individuals have been correctly reclassified from Intermediate Risk (IR) to Low Risk (LR) or High Risk (HR). That is, the actual event rates in these reclassified groups, whose risks as calculated by the Framingham algorithm put them in the IR risk range, were either lower or higher than this range once coronary calcification was factored in. This is taken as evidence in favor of coronary calcification to measure risk. And it is.

But it is also evidence that the range of risk for subgroups of individuals may fall outside the boundaries of the estimated risk for the total group. That is, the range of risks for the group as estimated by the confidence intervals does not cover the range of risks for all the individuals within that group. Put differently, whatever estimate of risk the algorithm produces for any individual, the confidence intervals for that prediction are much broader than we imagine. The conclusion that follows is that we must be skeptical of the accuracy for the individual of the risk estimate that is produced by any of the conventional algorithms. The individual who is at calculated Intermediate Risk may be at Intermediate Risk but there is also a far from negligible chance that they are at High or Low Risk. Accordingly, if our objective is to treat groups of subjects, the estimate is acceptable but if our objective is to give the best care to the individuals within groups, it is not.

7.3.4 How Age Makes the Concept of Risk Virtually Meaningless

The purpose of any risk algorithm is to separate out within a larger group those who need medical attention from those who do not. However, when the portion of those at high risk becomes large enough, separation no longer matters. If everyone is at high risk, estimating risk no longer matters. As shown above, the AHA/ACC guidelines have virtually achieved this result.[254] Over the age of 60, 90% of men are eligible for prevention. And most of the rest are so close to the boundary that for practical purposes, the algorithm designates everyone as eligible for therapy. Indeed, even those without any risk factors for CVD are included. Thus any white male with no risk factors for CVD – that is, a non-smoker, non-diabetic with a normal blood pressure and a normal non-HDL-C – will exceed the calculated 7.5% 10-year risk of a cardiovascular event at age 63 as will be the case for a 66-year-old African American man, a 70-year-old African American woman or a 71-year-old white woman. If everyone is at high risk, separation is irrelevant and preventive statin therapy should be initiated based on age alone.

When Wald and Law argued for age 50 as the initiation point of universal therapy,[232] this was their point, an argument that was not accepted at the time but without attribution and with a decade added onto the cut point, has become the conventional recommendation.[223] Of course, different countries and different guideline groups set the barrier differently. Nevertheless, once the portion of those eligible for prevention becomes high enough, the imprecision in allocation is taken into account, the inevitable change in risk with age alone, the distinction between those selected for therapy and those who are not become less and less meaningful. The disadvantages are that everyone will be exposed to the potential for side effects from the medications that will be given and not everyone will benefit from them and prevention will focus on those who are older and who will benefit less and ignore those who are younger and will benefit more.

7.4 The Causal Exposure Paradigm of Vascular Disease

It takes decades for the causes of disease to produce the complex lesions within the arteries that immediately antedate the clinical events (*see Figure 7.1*). The Causal Exposure paradigm calls for intervention against the causes of disease when they are identified, well before arterial disease has become advanced and events are imminent. The objective is to prevent the anatomic disease that is the essential precondition for the clinical events. Amongst the most powerful arguments for our position is that while we know much about what causes disease within arteries and while we have multiple proven therapies to interdict their malign effects within the arterial wall, we know little about what suddenly and irretrievably tips the complex interplay of healing and destructive forces within the arterial wall towards a clinical event. We know that statin-induced LDL lowering can substantially reduce, but far from eliminate, the likelihood of such an event. We know also that there are multiple pathological mechanisms that can produce sustained reductions in arterial flow. Given how many and how different they are, it seems unlikely that all will be preventable with LDL-lowering therapy. Indeed, statins prevent only the minority of events in all the clinical trials. To be sure, even late in the process, statin therapy produces substantial benefit but were it started earlier the benefits would be even more substantial. That is our hypothesis.

7.4.1 Risk and Benefit Relate to the Level of LDL

We submit there is much evidence against the view that seems to be so strongly held by all the guidelines that the benefits of statin therapy do not relate to the starting level of LDL and to the extent to which LDL is lowered from this level. We discussed this evidence extensively in the previous chapter on therapy (*Chapter 6*). Here, we will repeat only the most important points. The CTT meta-analysis,[230] and HPS[252] have been the two most influential analyses of the clinical benefits of statin therapy and the conclusion the authors and others have drawn is that the benefit of lowering LDL is determined by baseline risk and is not related to the level of LDL. As outlined above, this finding is indeed true for groups but only because the level of risk within the groups, particularly those without known vascular disease, is so variable. Since we treat individuals, not groups, we should be aware of the error of assuming the risk of a group is the same as the risk of any particular member of the group.

CTT[230] and HPS[252] have demonstrated that for each 1 mmol/l lowering of LDL-C, cardiovascular risk is reduced by approximately 20%. If clinical events are indeed reduced by 20% for each mmol reduction of LDL-C, the potential for benefit for an individual is related to their baseline level of LDL-C. Thus, if the target is an LDL-C of 2 mmol/l a patient with an LDL-C of 5 mmol/L has 3 potential units of decrease compared to a patient with a baseline level of LDL-C of only 3 mmol/l who has only 1.

If the initial event rate in both is the same, that rate will be reduced by 49% in the first patient but by only 20% in the second. (Figure 7.4) Moreover, the higher the LDL-C, the greater the absolute reduction in LDL-C with a given dose of a statin[232] and, therefore, the greater the benefit there will be from a given dose of a statin. Put simply, the worse the problem, the greater the gain.

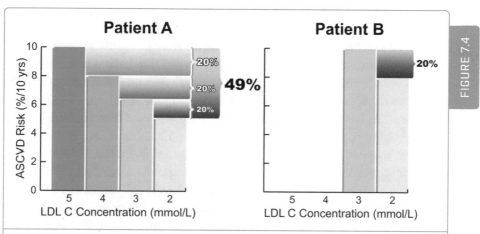

FIGURE 7.4

Two patients are illustrated, both at the same group risk of 100 events per unit time. In patient A on the left, reduction in LDL-C from 5 to 4 mmol will reduce clinical events by 20%. Therefore, if the baseline event rate is 100, it will be reduced to 80. Reduction from an LDL-C of 4 to 3 mmol/l will reduce the event rate by a further 20% decreasing it from 80 to 64. Decreasing from 3 to 2 mmol/l will reduce the event rate to 51.2 – a total decrease, therefore of 49%. By contrast, in patient B on the right, decreasing the LDL-C from 3 to 2 mmol/l will only decrease the event by 20% – in this case, from 100 to 80.

The second point is that the absolute reduction in LDL induced by a given dose of a given statin relates to the starting level of LDL: the higher the starting level, the greater the decrease. The relative potency of the statins is measured by the percent decrease in LDL-C or non-HDL-C or apoB induced by a given dose of a given statin. Atorvastatin 80 mg will reduce LDL-C by approximately 50%. Accordingly, the higher the starting level, the greater the absolute decrease; the greater the absolute decrease, the greater the clinical benefit that should result. Thus, 80 mg of atorvastatin will reduce an LDL-C of 2 mmol/l to 1 mmol/l with a reduction in events of 20% whereas the same dose of the same drug will reduce an LDL-C of 4 mmol/l to 2 mmol/l with a reduction in events of approximately 40%. Moreover, we must not forget that there is considerable individual variance in the response to a dose of a statin. Indeed, this is precisely the reason we believe the response to a statin should be carefully measured and the dose adjusted accordingly.

Thus, while the relative benefit may be the same, the absolute benefit of statin therapy will be greater in those with higher baseline LDL-C than in those with lower baseline LDL-C. It follows that while there is a continuous relation between LDL and risk, the absolute change and therefore the absolute clinical gain becomes smaller and smaller as the level of LDL becomes lower and lower.

7.4.2 Selection of Subjects for Earlier LDL-Lowering Therapy

We suggest that this decision be based on two criteria: the estimated 30-year risk of a coronary event and evidence of elevated LDL. By definition, the subjects to be considered for earlier intervention would be at levels of 10-year risk that are less than the Guidelines would recommend intervention. Such subjects would typically be 40 years of age or more, but less than 60 years of age. Their 30-year risk would be calculated as suggested by Pencina et al.[259] The choice of cut point is, as always, arbitrary but a value ≥ 20% should prompt consideration of further action. Evidence of elevated LDL should be sought. ApoB should be measured since approximately 20% of those with elevated non-HDL-C or LDL-C have cholesterol-enriched apoB particles and are not at increased medium- and long-term risk. This cannot be recognized if only LDL-C or non-HDL-C are measured. Evidence of persistent elevation of LDL-C or non-HDL-C or apoB should also be sought as we have shown, for example, that persistent, as opposed to intermittent elevation of non-HDL-C identifies a subgroup at particularly high cardiovascular risk over the next 20 years.[260]

7.4.3 Limitation of the Causal Exposure Paradigm

The critical limitation in our argument is evidence: no randomized clinical trial has been done or will ever be done to test whether earlier prevention will be more effective than later prevention. Moreover, no therapy is free of cost and statin therapy is no exception. The most significant risk to consider for early initiation of statin therapy is the risk of inducing diabetes. This risk appears to be low and confined to those who were already at high risk of this metabolic complication.

Summary

The risk paradigm presently governs cardiovascular prevention. However, because risk can only be high when anatomic intramural disease is extensive and advanced, the benefits of prevention will be limited. We believe that earlier treatment of causal factors such as LDL would produce better overall results since only some of the pathophysiological mechanisms that produce cardiovascular events are likely to be inhibited by statin therapy and if we prevent the disease, we will not have to be concerned about risk.

Appendix

Population distribution of LDL-C, non-HDL-C and apoB in the NHANES database (www.cdc.gov/nchs/nhanes)

Different guideline LDL-C targets are in green, non-HDL-C targets are in orange and apoB targets are in blue (see table 6.1 Chapter 6). Our targets for apoB are in red: moderate and high risk apoB < 0.75 g/l and very high risk apoB < 0.65 g/l.

Percentile	LDLC Mg/dl	LDLC Mmol/l	NonHDLC Mg/dl	NonHDLC Mmol/l	ApoB g/l
1	22	0,57	32	0,83	0,24
2	48	1,24	63	1,63	0,43
3	54	1,40	72	1,86	0,49
4	60	1,55	77	1,99	0,52
5	63	1,63	80	2,07	0,54
6	67	1,74	83	2,15	0,57
7	69	1,79	86	2,23	0,58
8	71	1,84	88	2,28	0,59
9	73	1,89	91	2,36	0,61
10	74	1,92	92	2,38	0,62
11	76	1,97	94	2,43	0,63
12	77	1,99	96	2,49	0,64
13	79	2,05	98	2,54	0,65
14	80	2,07	99	2,56	
15	81	2,10	101	2,62	0,66
16	83	2,15			0,67
17	84	2,18	103	2,67	0,68
18	85	2,20	105	2,72	0,69
19	86	2,23	106	2,75	0,70
20	87	2,25	107	2,77	
21	88	2,28	108	2,80	0,71
22	90	2,33	109	2,82	0,72
23			110	2,85	0,73
24	91	2,36	111	2,87	
25					0,74

Percentile	LDLC Mg/dl	LDLC Mmol/l	NonHDLC Mg/dl	NonHDLC Mmol/l	ApoB g/l
26	93	2,41	113	2,93	0,75
27	94	2,43	115	2,98	
28	95	2,46			0,76
29	96	2,49	116	3,00	
30	97	2,51	118	3,06	0,77
31	98	2,54	119	3,08	0,78
32	99	2,56	120	3,11	
33	100	2,59	121	3,13	0,79
34	101	2,62	122	3,16	
35	102	2,64	123	3,19	0,80
36	103	2,67	124	3,21	0,81
37			125	3,24	
38	104	2,69	126	3,26	0,82
39			127	3,29	0,83
40	106	2,75	128	3,32	
41	107	2,77			0,84
42	108	2,80	130	3,37	0,85
43	109	2,82	132	3,42	
44			133	3,44	0,86
45	110	2,85			
46	111	2,87	134	3,47	0,87
47	112	2,90	135	3,50	
48			136	3,52	0,88
49	113	2,93	137	3,55	0,89
50	114	2,95	138	3,57	
51	115	2,98	139	3,60	0,90
52	116	3,00	140	3,63	
53	117	3,03	141	3,65	0,91
54	118	3,06	142	3,68	
55	119	3,08	143	3,70	0,92
56					0,93
57	120	3,11	144	3,73	
58	121	3,13	145	3,76	0,94
59	122	3,16	146	3,78	
60	123	3,19	147	3,81	0,95
61	124	3,21	148	3,83	0,96
62	125	3,24	149	3,86	
63	126	3,26	150	3,89	0,97

Percentile	LDLC Mg/dl	LDLC Mmol/l	NonHDLC Mg/dl	NonHDLC Mmol/l	ApoB g/l
64	127	3,29	151	3,91	0,00
65	128	3,32	152	3,94	
66			153	3,96	0,99
67	129	3,34	154	3,99	1,00
68	130	3,37	156	4,04	1,01
69	131	3,39	157	4,07	
70	132	3,42	158	4,09	1,02
71	133	3,44	159	4,12	
72	134	3,47	160	4,14	1,03
73	135	3,50	161	4,17	1,04
74	136	3,52	163	4,22	1,05
75	137	3,55	164	4,25	1,06
76	138	3,57	165	4,27	
77	139	3,60	167	4,33	1,07
78	140	3,63	168	4,35	1,08
79	142	3,68	169	4,38	1,09
80	143	3,70	170	4,40	1,10
81	144	3,73	172	4,45	
82	146	3,78	173	4,48	1,11
83	147	3,81	175	4,53	1,13
84	148	3,83	177	4,58	1,14
85	150	3,89	179	4,64	1,15
86	152	3,94	181	4,69	1,16
87	153	3,96	183	4,74	1,17
88	155	4,01	186	4,82	1,18
89	157	4,07	188	4,87	1,20
90	160	4,14	191	4,95	1,21
91	162	4,20	193	5,00	1,22
92	165	4,27	195	5,05	1,24
93	167	4,33	198	5,13	1,26
94	170	4,40	202	5,23	1,27
95	175	4,53	205	5,31	1,29
96	178	4,61	209	5,41	1,31
97	182	4,71	215	5,57	1,34
98	188	4,87	220	5,70	1,39
99	194	5,02	228	5,91	1,45
100	209	5,41	246	6,37	1,53

References

1. Kwiterovich, P.O. *The John Hopkins Textbook of Dyslipidemia.* (Lippincott Williams & Wilkins, 2012).
2. Choi, B.G., Badimon, J.J., Moreno, P.R. & Fuster, V. in: *Clinical Lipidology, A companion to Braunwald's Heart Disease* (Ballantyne, C.M.) (2009).
3. Pownall, H.J. & Gotto, A.M., Jr. Human Plasma Lipoprotein Metabolism in: *Clinical Lipidology, A companion to Braunwald's Heart Disease* (Ballantyne, C.M.) (2009).
4. Fazio, S. & Linton, M.F. in: *Clinical Lipidology, A companion to Braunwald's Heart Disease* (Ballantyne, C.M.) (2009).
5. Brewer, H.B., Gregg, R.E., Hoeg, J.M. & Fojo, S.S. Apolipoproteins and lipoproteins in human plasma: an overview. *Clin Chem.* **34,** B4-8 (1988).
6. Teng, B., Burant, C.F. & Davidson, N.O. Molecular cloning of an apolipoprotein B messenger RNA editing protein. *Science.* **260,** 1816-1819 (1993).
7. Sacks, F.M. The crucial roles of apolipoproteins E and C-III in apoB lipoprotein metabolism in normolipidemia and hypertriglyceridemia. *Curr Opin Lipidol.* **26,** 56-63 (2015).
8. Zheng, C. Updates on apolipoprotein CIII: fulfilling promise as a therapeutic target for hypertriglyceridemia and cardiovascular disease. *Curr Opin Lipidol.* **25,** 35-39 (2014).
9. Segrest, J.P., Jackson, R.L., Morrisett, J.D. & Gotto, A.M. A molecular theory of lipid-protein interactions in the plasma lipoproteins. *FEBS Lett.* **38,** 247-258 (1974).
10. Sniderman, A.D., Cianflone, K., Arner, P., Summers, L.K. & Frayn, K.N. The adipocyte, fatty acid trapping, and atherogenesis. *Arterioscler Thromb Vasc Biol.* **18,** 147-151 (1998).
11. Beisiegel, U., Weber, W., Ihrke, G., Herz, J. & Stanley, K.K. The LDL-receptor-related protein, LRP, is an apolipoprotein E-binding protein. *Nature.* **341,** 162-164 (1989).
12. Fisher, E., Lake, E. & McLeod, R.S. Apolipoprotein B100 quality control and the regulation of hepatic very low density lipoprotein secretion. *J Biomed Res.* **28,** 178-193 (2014).
13. Sparks, J.D., Sparks, C.E. & Adeli, K. Selective hepatic insulin resistance, VLDL overproduction, and hypertriglyceridemia. *Arterioscler Thromb Vasc Biol.* **32,** 2104-2112 (2012).
14. Olofsson, S.-O. & Borén, J. Apolipoprotein B secretory regulation by degradation. *Arterioscler Thromb Vasc Biol.* **32,** 1334-1338 (2012).
15. Fisher, E.A. The degradation of apolipoprotein B100: multiple opportunities to regulate VLDL triglyceride production by different proteolytic pathways. *Biochim Biophys Acta.* **1821,** 778-781 (2012).
16. Xiang, S.Q., Cianflone, K., Kalant, D. & Sniderman, A.D. Differential binding of triglyceride-rich lipoproteins to lipoprotein lipase. *J Lipid Res.* **40,** 1655-1663 (1999).
17. Sniderman, A.D., de Graaf, J., Couture, P. *et al.* Regulation of plasma LDL: the apoB paradigm. *Clin Sci.* **118,** 333-339 (2010).

18. Emerging Risk Factors Collaboration *et al*. Lipoprotein(a) concentration and the risk of coronary heart disease, stroke, and nonvascular mortality. JAMA. **302,** 412-423 (2009).

19. Kamstrup, P.R., Tybjaerg-Hansen, A., Steffensen, R. & Nordestgaard, B.G. Genetically elevated lipoprotein(a) and increased risk of myocardial infarction. JAMA. **301,** 2331-2339 (2009).

20. Clarke, R., Peden J.F., Hopewell, J.C. *et al*. Genetic variants associated with Lp(a) lipoprotein level and coronary disease. N Engl J Med. **361,** 2518-2528 (2009).

21. Thanassoulis, G., Campbell, C.Y., Owens, D.S. *et al*. Genetic associations with valvular calcification and aortic stenosis. N Engl J Med. **368,** 503-512 (2013).

22. AIM-HIGH Investigators *et al*. Niacin in patients with low HDL cholesterol levels receiving intensive statin therapy. N Engl J Med. **365,** 2255-2267 (2011).

23. Packard, C.J., Munro, A., Lorimer, A.R., Gotto, A.M. & Shepherd, J. Metabolism of apolipoprotein B in large triglyceride-rich very low density lipoproteins of normal and hypertriglyceridemic subjects. J Clin Invest. **74,** 2178-2192 (1984).

24. Boren, J., Taskinen, M.R. & Adiels, M. Kinetic studies to investigate lipoprotein metabolism. J Intern Med. **271,** 166-173 (2012).

25. Hopkins, P.N., Brinton, E.A. & Nanjee, M.N. Hyperlipoproteinemia type 3: the forgotten phenotype. Curr Atheroscler Rep. **16,** 440-19 (2014).

26. Marais, A.D., Solomon, G.A.E. & Blom, D.J. Dysbetalipoproteinaemia: a mixed hyperlipidaemia of remnant lipoproteins due to mutations in apolipoprotein E. Crit Rev Clin Lab Sci. **51,** 46-62 (2014).

27. Nordestgaard, B.G. & Tybjaerg-Hansen, A. IDL, VLDL, chylomicrons and atherosclerosis. Eur J Epidemiol. **8 Suppl 1,** 92-98 (1992).

28. Mahley, R.W. Atherogenic lipoproteins and coronary artery disease: concepts derived from recent advances in cellular and molecular biology. Circulation. **72,** 943-948 (1985).

29. Barter, P.J., Ballantyne, C.M., Carmena, R., *et al*. Apo B versus cholesterol in estimating cardiovascular risk and in guiding therapy: report of the thirty-person/ten-country panel. J Intern Med. **259,** 247-258 (2006).

30. Packard, C.J., Demant, T., Stewart, J.P., *et al*. Apolipoprotein B metabolism and the distribution of VLDL and LDL subfractions. J Lipid Res. **41,** 305-318 (2000).

31. Sniderman, A.D., Scantlebury, T. & Cianflone, K. Hypertriglyceridemic hyperapob: the unappreciated atherogenic dyslipoproteinemia in type 2 diabetes mellitus. Ann Intern Med. **135,** 447-459 (2001).

32. Grundy, S.M., Vega, G.L., Tomassini, J.E. & Tershakovec, A.M. Comparisons of apolipoprotein B levels estimated by immunoassay, nuclear magnetic resonance, vertical auto profile, and non-high-density lipoprotein cholesterol in subjects with hypertriglyceridemia (SAFARI Trial). Am J Cardiol. **108,** 40-46 (2011).

33. Krauss, R.M. All low-density lipoprotein particles are not created equal. Arterioscler Thromb Vasc Biol. **34,** 959-961 (2014).

34. Krauss, R.M. & Burke, D. J. Identification of multiple subclasses of plasma low density lipoproteins in normal humans. J Lipid Res. **23,** 97-104 (1982).

35. Berneis, K.K. & Krauss, R.M. Metabolic origins and clinical significance of LDL heterogeneity. J Lipid Res. **43,** 1363-1379 (2002).

36. de Graaf, J., Hak-Lemmers, H.L., Hectors, M.P. *et al*. Enhanced susceptibility to in vitro oxidation of the dense low density lipoprotein subfraction in healthy subjects. Arterioscler Thromb. **11,** 298-306 (1991).

37. Tremblay, A.J., Sniderman, A.D., Gagné, C., Bergeron, J. & Couture, P. Differential impact of plasma triglycerides on HDL-cholesterol and HDL-apo A-I in a large cohort. Clin Biochem. **40,** 25-29 (2007).

38. Lamarche, B., Uffelman, K.D., Carpentier, A. *et al.* Triglyceride enrichment of HDL enhances in vivo metabolic clearance of HDL apo A-I in healthy men. *J Clin Invest.* **103,** 1191-1199 (1999).

39. Gofman, J.W. & Lindgren, F. The role of lipids and lipoproteins in atherosclerosis. *Science.* **111,** 166-171 (1950).

40. Sniderman, A.D. & Cianflone, K. Metabolic disruptions in the adipocyte-hepatocyte fatty acid axis as causes of HyperapoB. *Int J Obes Relat Metab Disord.* **19 Suppl 1,** S27-33 (1995).

41. Sniderman, A.D. & Cianflone, K. Substrate delivery as a determinant of hepatic apoB secretion. *Arterioscler Thromb.* **13,** 629-636 (1993).

42. Cianflone, K.M., Yasruel, Z., Rodriguez, M.A., Vas, D. & Sniderman, A.D. Regulation of apoB secretion from HepG2 cells: evidence for a critical role for cholesteryl ester synthesis in the response to a fatty acid challenge. *J Lipid Res.* **31,** 2045-2055 (1990).

43. Faraj, M., Sniderman, A.D. & Cianflone, K. ASP enhances in situ lipoprotein lipase activity by increasing fatty acid trapping in adipocytes. *J Lipid Res.* **45,** 657-666 (2004).

44. Merkel, M., Eckel, R.H. & Goldberg, I.J. Lipoprotein lipase: genetics, lipid uptake, and regulation. *J Lipid Res.* **43,** 1997-2006 (2002).

45. Frayn, K.N. Adipose tissue as a buffer for daily lipid flux. *Diabetologia.* **45,** 1201-1210 (2002).

46. Karpe, F., Dickmann, J.R. & Frayn, K.N. Fatty acids, obesity, and insulin resistance: time for a reevaluation. *Diabetes.* **60,** 2441-2449 (2011).

47. Romacho, T., Elsen, M., Röhrborn, D. & Eckel, J. Adipose tissue and its role in organ crosstalk. *Acta Physiol (Oxf).* **210,** 733-753 (2014).

48. Cianflone, K., Xia, Z. & Chen, L.Y. Critical review of acylation-stimulating protein physiology in humans and rodents. *Biochim Biophys Acta.* **1609,** 127-143 (2003).

49. MacLaren, R., Cui, W. & Cianflone, K. Adipokines and the immune system: an adipocentric view. *Adv Exp Med Biol.* **632,** 1-21 (2008).

50. Andersson, D.P., Löfgren, P., Thorell, A., Arner, P. & Hoffstedt, J. Visceral fat cell lipolysis and cardiovascular risk factors in obesity. *Horm Metab Res.* **43,** 809-815 (2011).

51. Sniderman, A.D., Cianflone, K., Summers, L., Fielding, B. & Frayn, K. The acylation-stimulating protein pathway and regulation of postprandial metabolism. *Proc Nutr Soc.* **56,** 703-712 (1997).

52. Sniderman, A.D., Cianflone, K. & Frayn, K. The pathogenetic role of impaired fatty acid trapping by adipocytes in generating the pleiotropic features of hyperapoB. *Diabetologia.* **40 Suppl 2,** S152-4 (1997).

53. Smith, J., Al-Amri, M., Dorairaj, P. & Sniderman, A. The adipocyte life cycle hypothesis. *Clin Sci.* **110,** 1-9 (2006).

54. Sniderman A.D., Bhopal, R., Prabhakaran D. Why might Asians be so susceptible to central obesity and its atherogenic consequences? The adipose tissue overflow hypothesis. *Int J Epidemiol.* **36,** 220-225 (2007).

55. Laurencikiene, J., Skurk, T., Kulyté, A. *et al.* Regulation of lipolysis in small and large fat cells of the same subject. *J Clin Endocrinol Metab.* **96,** E2045-9 (2011).

56. Heinonen, S., Saarinen, L., Naukkarinen, J. *et al.* Adipocyte morphology and implications for metabolic derangements in acquired obesity. *Int J Obes (Lond).* **38,** 1423-1431 (2014).

57. Lear, S.A., Kohli, S., Bondy, G.P., Tchernof, A. & Sniderman, A.D. Ethnic variation in fat and lean body mass and the association with insulin resistance. *J. Clin Endocrinol Metab.* **94,** 4696-4702 (2009).

58. Kohli, S., Sniderman, A.D., Tchernof, A. & Lear, S.A. Ethnic-specific differences in abdominal subcutaneous adipose tissue compartments. *Obesity.* **18,** 2177-2183 (2010).

59. Parlee, S.D., Lentz, S.I., Mori, H. & MacDougald, O.A. Quantifying size and number of adipocytes in adipose tissue. *Meth Enzymol.* **537,** 93-122 (2014).

60. Hodson, L. & Frayn, K.N. Hepatic fatty acid partitioning. *Curr Opin Lipidol.* **22,** 216-224 (2011).

61. Zhang, Z., Cianflone, K. & Sniderman, A.D. Role of cholesterol ester mass in regulation of secretion of ApoB100 lipoprotein particles by hamster hepatocytes and effects of statins on that relationship. *Arterioscler Thromb Vasc Biol.* **19**, 743-752 (1999).

62. Sniderman, A.D., Thanassoulis, G., Couture, P., *et al.* Hepatic cholesterol homeostasis: is the low-density lipoprotein pathway a regulatory or a shunt pathway? *Arterioscler Thromb Vasc Biol.* **33**, 2481-2490 (2013).

63. Brown, M.S. & Goldstein, J. L. A receptor-mediated pathway for cholesterol homeostasis. *Science.* **232**, 34-47 (1986).

64. Sniderman, A.D., Tsimikas, S. & Fazio, S. The severe hypercholesterolemia phenotype: clinical diagnosis, management, and emerging therapies. *J Am Coll Cardiol.* **63**, 1935-1947 (2014).

65. Sniderman, A.D., Zhang, X.J. & Cianflone, K. Governance of the concentration of plasma LDL: a reevaluation of the LDL receptor paradigm. *Atherosclerosis.* **148**, 215-229 (2000).

66. Sniderman, A.D., Dagenais, G.R., Cantin, B., Després, J.P. & Lamarche, B. High apolipoprotein B with low high-density lipoprotein cholesterol and normal plasma triglycerides and cholesterol. *Am J Cardiol.* **87**, 792-3-A8 (2001).

67. Sniderman, A.D., Zhang, Z., Genest, J. & Cianflone, K. Effects on apoB-100 secretion and bile acid synthesis by redirecting cholesterol efflux from HepG2 cells. *J Lipid Res.* **44**, 527-532 (2003).

68. Kozarsky, K.F., Donahee, M.H., Rigotti, A., *et al.* Overexpression of the HDL receptor SR-BI alters plasma HDL and bile cholesterol levels. *Nature.* **387**, 414-417 (1997).

69. Ji, Y., Wang, N., Ramakrishnan, R., *et al.* Hepatic scavenger receptor BI promotes rapid clearance of high density lipoprotein free cholesterol and its transport into bile. *J Biol Chem.* **274**, 33398-33402 (1999).

70. Yuan, Q., Bie, J., Wang, J., Ghosh, S.S. & Ghosh, S. Cooperation between hepatic cholesteryl ester hydrolase and scavenger receptor BI for hydrolysis of HDL-CE. *J Lipid Res.* **54**, 3078-3084 (2013).

71. Tiwari, S. & Siddiqi, S.A. Intracellular trafficking and secretion of VLDL. *Arterioscler Thromb Vasc Biol.* **32**, 1079-1086 (2012).

72. Adiels, M., Borén, J., Caslake, M.J, *et al.* Overproduction of VLDL1 driven by hyperglycemia is a dominant feature of diabetic dyslipidemia. *Arterioscler Thromb Vasc Biol.* **25**, 1697-1703 (2005).

73. Chait, A., Albers, J.J. & Brunzell, J.D. Very low density lipoprotein overproduction in genetic forms of hypertriglyceridaemia. *Eur J Clin Invest.* **10**, 17-22 (1980).

74. Teng, B., Sniderman, A.D., Soutar, A.K. & Thompson, G.R. Metabolic basis of hyperapobetalipoproteinemia. Turnover of apolipoprotein B in low density lipoprotein and its precursors and subfractions compared with normal and familial hypercholesterolemia. *J Clin Invest.* **77**, 663-672 (1986).

75. Sniderman, A.D., Hogue, J.-C., Bergeron, J., Gagné, C. & Couture, P. Non-HDL cholesterol and apoB in dyslipidaemia. *Clin Sci.* **114**, 149-155 (2008).

76. Sniderman, A.D., Zhang, Z. & Cianflone, K. Divergent responses of the liver to increased delivery of glucose or fatty acids: implications for the pathogenesis of type IV hyperlipoproteinemia. *Atherosclerosis.* **137**, 291-301 (1998).

77. Fredrickson, D.S., Levy, R.I. & Lees, R.S. Fat transport in lipoproteins – an integrated approach to mechanisms and disorders. *N Engl J Med.* **276**, 273-81 concl (1967).

78. Fredrickson, D.S., Levy, R.I. & Lees, R.S. Fat transport in lipoproteins – an integrated approach to mechanisms and disorders. *N Engl J Med.* **276**, 215-25 contd (1967).

79. Fredrickson, D.S., Levy, R.I. & Lees, R.S. Fat transport in lipoproteins – an integrated approach to mechanisms and disorders. *N Engl J Med.* **276**, 148-56 contd (1967).

80. Fredrickson, D.S., Levy, R.I. & Lees, R.S. Fat transport in lipoproteins – an integrated approach to mechanisms and disorders. *N Engl J Med.* **276**, 94-103 contd (1967).

81. Fredrickson, D.S., Levy, R.I. & Lees, R.S. Fat transport in lipoproteins – an integrated approach to mechanisms and disorders. *N Engl J Med.* **276**, 34-42 contd (1967).

82. Sniderman, A., Couture, P. & De Graaf, J. Diagnosis and treatment of apolipoprotein B dys-lipoproteinemias. *Nat Rev Endocrinol.* **6,** 335-346 (2010).

83. De Graaf, J., Couture, P. & Sniderman, A. A diagnostic algorithm for the atherogenic apolipo-protein B dyslipoproteinemias. *Nat Clin Pract Endocrinol Metab.* **4,** 608-618 (2008).

84. de Nijs, T., Sniderman, A. & De Graaf, J. ApoB versus non-HDL-cholesterol: diagnosis and car-diovascular risk management. *Crit Rev Clin Lab Sci.* **50,** 163-171 (2013).

85. Sniderman, A.D. Applying apoB to the diagnosis and therapy of the atherogenic dyslipopro-teinemias: a clinical diagnostic algorithm. *Curr Opin Lipidol.* **15,** 433-438 (2004).

86. Brook, R.D., Doshi, H., Bard, R.L. & Rubenfire, M. Potential effect of an apoprotein B-based algorithm on management of new patients with hypertriglyceridemia referred to a specialty lipid clinic. *Clin Cardiol.* **32,** 251-255 (2009).

87. Holewijn, S., Sniderman, A.D., den Heijer, M. *et al.* Application and validation of a diagnostic algorithm for the atherogenic apoB dyslipoproteinemias: ApoB dyslipoproteinemias in a Dutch population-based study. *Eur J Clin Invest.* **41,** 423-433 (2011).

88. Sniderman, A., Tremblay, A., Bergeron, J., Gagné, C. & Couture, P. Diagnosis of type III hyper-lipoproteinemia from plasma total cholesterol, triglyceride, and apolipoprotein B. *J Clin Lipidol.* **1,** 256-263 (2007).

89. Sniderman, A.D., Lamarche, B., Tilley, J., Seccombe, D. & Frohlich, J. Hypertriglyceridemic hy-perapoB in type 2 diabetes. *Diabetes Care.* **25,** 579-582 (2002).

90. Wang, H. & Eckel, R. H. Lipoprotein lipase: from gene to obesity. *Am J Physiol Endocrinol Metab.* **297,** E271-88 (2009).

91. Miller, M., Stone, N.J., Ballantyne, C. *et al.* Triglycerides and cardiovascular disease: a scientific statement from the American Heart Association. *Circulation.* **123,** 2292-2333 (2011).

92. Brown, W.V., Brunzell, J.D., Eckel, R.H. & Stone, N.J. Severe hypertriglyceridemia. *J Clin Lipidol.* **6,** 397-408 (2012).

93. Chokshi, N., Blumenschein, S.D., Ahmad, Z. & Garg, A. Genotype-phenotype relationships in patients with type 1 hyperlipoproteinemia. *J Clin Lipidol.* **8,** 287-295 (2014).

94. Johansen, C.T. & Hegele, R. A. Genetic bases of hypertriglyceridemic phenotypes. *Curr Opin Lipidol.* **22,** 247-253 (2011).

95. Beigneux, A.P. *et al.* GPIHBP1 Missense Mutations Often Cause Multimerization of GPIHBP1 and Thereby Prevent Lipoprotein Lipase Binding. *Circ. Res.* 114.305085 (2014).

96. Nilsson, S.K., Heeren, J., Olivecrona, G. & Merkel, M. Apolipoprotein A-V; a potent triglyceride reducer. *Atherosclerosis.* **219,** 15-21 (2011).

97. Tremblay, A.J., Lamarche, B., Labonté, M.È. *et al.* Dietary medium-chain triglyceride supplemen-tation has no effect on apolipoprotein B-48 and apolipoprotein B-100 kinetics in insulin-resistant men. *Am J Clin Nutr.* **99,** 54-61 (2014).

98. Kastelein, J.J.P., Maki, K.C., Susekov, A. *et al.* Omega-3 free fatty acids for the treatment of severe hypertriglyceridemia: the EpanoVa fOr Lowering Very high triglyceridEs (EVOLVE) trial. *J Clin Lipidol.* **8,** 94-106 (2014).

99. Gaudet, D., Brisson, D., Tremblay, K. *et al.* Targeting APOC3 in the familial chylomicronemia syndrome. *N Engl J Med.* **371,** 2200-2206 (2014).

100. Gaudet, D. *et al.* Efficacy and long-term safety of alipogene tiparvovec (AAV1-LPLS447X) gene therapy for lipoprotein lipase deficiency: an open-label trial. *Gene Ther.* **20,** 361-369 (2013).

101. Sacks, F.M., Stanesa, M. & Hegele, R.A. Severe hypertriglyceridemia with pancreatitis: thirteen years' treatment with lomitapide. *JAMA.* **174,** 443-447 (2014).

102. Morganroth, J., Levy, R.I. & Fredrickson, D.S. The biochemical, clinical, and genetic features of type III hyperlipoproteinemia. *Ann Intern Med.* **82,** 158-174 (1975).

103. Connelly, P.W. & Hegele, R.A. Hepatic lipase deficiency. *Crit Rev Clin Lab Sci* **35,** 547-572 (1998).

104. Angelin, B., Hershon, K.S. & Brunzell, J.D. Bile acid metabolism in hereditary forms of hypertriglyceridemia: evidence for an increased synthesis rate in monogenic familial hypertriglyceridemia. *Proc Natl Acad Sci U.S.A.* **84,** 5434-5438 (1987).

105. Ooi, E.M.M., Russell, B.S., Olson, E. *et al.* Apolipoprotein B-100-containing lipoprotein metabolism in subjects with lipoprotein lipase gene mutations. *Arterioscler Thromb Vasc Biol.* **32,** 459-466 (2012).

106. Dorfmeister, B. *et al.* Effects of six APOA5 variants, identified in patients with severe hypertriglyceridemia, on in vitro lipoprotein lipase activity and receptor binding. *Arterioscler Thromb Vasc Biol.* **28,** 1866-1871 (2008).

107. Goldstein, J.L., Schrott, H.G., Hazzard, W.R., Bierman, E.L. & Motulsky, A.G. Hyperlipidemia in Coronary Heart Disease II. Genetic analysis of lipid levels in 176 families and delineation of a new inherited disorder, combined hyperlipidemia. *J. Clin. Invest.* **52,** 1544-1568 (1973).

108. Nikkilä, E.A. & Aro, A. Family study of serum lipids and lipoproteins in coronary heart-disease. *Lancet* **.1,** 954-959 (1973).

109. Rose, H.D. Recurrent illness following acute coxsackie B 4 myocarditis. *Am J Med.* **54,** 544-548 (1973).

110. Austin, M.A., McKnight, B, Edwards, K.L. *et al.* Cardiovascular disease mortality in familial forms of hypertriglyceridemia: A 20-year prospective study. *Circulation.* **101,** 2777-2782 (2000).

111. Brunzell, J.D., Schrott, H.G., Motulsky, A.G. & Bierman, E.L. Myocardial infarction in the familial forms of hypertriglyceridemia. *Metab Clin Exp.* **25,** 313-320 (1976).

112. Sniderman, A.D., Castro Cabezas, M., Ribalta, J. *et al.* A proposal to redefine familial combined hyperlipidaemia – third workshop on FCHL held in Barcelona from 3 to 5 May 2001, during the scientific sessions of the European Society for Clinical Investigation. in *Eur J Clin Invest.* **32,** 71-73 (2002).

113. Demacker, P.N.M., Veerkamp M.J., Bredie, S.J., *et al.* Comparison of the measurement of lipids and lipoproteins versus assay of apolipoprotein B for estimation of coronary heart disease risk: a study in familial combined hyperlipidemia. *Atherosclerosis.* **153,** 483-490 (2000).

114. Veerkamp, M.J., De Graaf, J., Hendriks, J.C.M., Demacker, P.N.M. & Stalenhoef, A.F.H. Nomogram to diagnose familial combined hyperlipidemia on the basis of results of a 5-year follow-up study. *Circulation.* **109,** 2980-2985 (2004).

115. Veerkamp, M.J., de Graaf, J., Bredie, S.J., *et al.* Diagnosis of familial combined hyperlipidemia based on lipid phenotype expression in 32 families: results of a 5-year follow-up study. *Arterioscler Thromb Vasc Biol.* **22,** 274-282 (2002).

116. Brunzell, J.D. *et al.* Plasma lipoproteins in familial combined hyperlipidemia and monogenic familial hypertriglyceridemia. *J Lipid Res.* **24,** 147-155 (1983).

117. van Greevenbroek, M.M.J., Stalenhoef, A.F.H., De Graaf, J. & Brouwers, M.C.G.J. Familial combined hyperlipidemia: from molecular insights to tailored therapy. *Curr Opin Lipidol.* **25,** 176-182 (2014).

118. ter Avest, E., Sniderman, A.D., Bredie, S.J. *et al.* Effect of aging and obesity on the expression of dyslipidaemia in children from families with familial combined hyperlipidaemia. *Clin Sci.* **112,** 131-139 (2007).

119. van der Kallen, C.J.H., Voors-Pette, C. & de Bruin, T.W.A. Abdominal obesity and expression of familial combined hyperlipidemia. *Obes Res.* **12,** 2054-2061 (2004).

120. Sniderman, A., Bailey, S.D. & Engert, J.C. Familial combined hyperlipidaemia: how can genetic disorders be common, complex and comprehensible? *Clin Sci.* **113,** 365-367 (2007).

121. De Graaf, J., Veerkamp, M.J. & Stalenhoef, A.F.H. Metabolic pathogenesis of familial combined hyperlipidaemia with emphasis on insulin resistance, adipose tissue metabolism and free fatty acids. *J R Soc Med.* **95 Suppl 42,** 46-53 (2002).

122. Rydén, M., Andersson, D.P., Bernard, S., Spalding, K. & Arner, P. Adipocyte triglyceride turnover and lipolysis in lean and overweight subjects. J Lipid Res. **54,** 2909-2913 (2013).

123. Frayn, K., Bernard, S., Spalding, K. & Arner, P. Adipocyte triglyceride turnover is independently associated with atherogenic dyslipidemia. J Am Heart Assoc. **1,** e003467-e003467 (2012).

124. Arner, P. et al. Dynamics of human adipose lipid turnover in health and metabolic disease. Nature. **478,** 110-113 (2011).

125. Veerkamp, M.J., de Graaf, J. & Stalenhoef, A.F.H. Role of insulin resistance in familial combined hyperlipidemia. Arterioscler Thromb Vasc Biol. **25,** 1026-1031 (2005).

126. van der Vleuten, G.M., Veerkamp, M.J., van Tits, L.J. et al. Elevated leptin levels in subjects with familial combined hyperlipidemia are associated with the increased risk for CVD. Atherosclerosis. **183,** 355-360 (2005).

127. van der Vleuten, G.M., van Tits, L.J., den Heijer, M. et al. Decreased adiponectin levels in familial combined hyperlipidemia patients contribute to the atherogenic lipid profile. J Lipid Res. **46,** 2398-2404 (2005).

128. van Greevenbroek, M.M.J., Ghosh, S., van der Kallen, C.J. et al. Up-regulation of the complement system in subcutaneous adipocytes from nonobese, hypertriglyceridemic subjects is associated with adipocyte insulin resistance. J Clin Endocrinol Metab. **97,** 4742-4752 (2012).

129. Horswell, S. D. et al. CDKN2B expression in adipose tissue of familial combined hyperlipidemia patients. J Lipid Res. **54,** 3491-3505 (2013).

130. Brouwers, M.C.G.J., van Greevenbroek, M.M.J., Stehouwer, C.D.A., De Graaf, J. & Stalenhoef, A.F.H. The genetics of familial combined hyperlipidaemia. Nat Rev Endocrinol. **8,** 352-362 (2012).

131. Auer, S. et al. Potential role of upstream stimulatory factor 1 gene variant in familial combined hyperlipidemia and related disorders. Arterioscler Thromb Vasc Biol. **32,** 1535-1544 (2012).

132. Rosenthal, E.A., Ranchalis, J., Crosslin, D.R. et al. Joint linkage and association analysis with exome sequence data implicates SLC25A40 in hypertriglyceridemia. Am J Hum Genet. **93,** 1035-1045 (2013).

133. Brouwers, M.C.G.J., Troutt, J.S., van Greevenbroek, M.M. et al. Plasma proprotein convertase subtilisin kexin type 9 is a heritable trait of familial combined hyperlipidaemia. Clin Sci. **121,** 397-403 (2011).

134. Chernogubova, E. et al. Common and low-frequency genetic variants in the PCSK9 locus influence circulating PCSK9 levels. Arterioscler Thromb Vasc Biol. **32,** 1526-1534 (2012).

135. Baila-Rueda, L. Mateo-Gallego, R., Jarauta, E., et al. Bile acid synthesis precursors in familial combined hyperlipidemia: The oxysterols 24S-hydroxycholesterol and 27-hydroxycholesterol. Biochem Biophys Res Commun. **446,** 731-735 (2014).

136. Lupattelli, G. Siepi, D., De Vuono, S. et al. Cholesterol metabolism differs after statin therapy according to the type of hyperlipemia. Life Sci. **90,** 846-850 (2012).

137. van Himbergen, T.M., Otokozawa S, Matthan NR et al. Familial combined hyperlipidemia is associated with alterations in the cholesterol synthesis pathway. Arterioscler Thromb Vasc Biol. **30,** 113-120 (2010).

138. Brouwers, M.C.G.J. et al. Plasma proprotein convertase subtilisin kexin type 9 levels are related to markers of cholesterol synthesis in familial combined hyperlipidemia. Nutr Metab Cardiovasc Dis **23,** 1115-1121 (2013).

139. ACCORD Study Group et al. Effects of combination lipid therapy in type 2 diabetes mellitus. N Engl J Med. **362,** 1563-1574 (2010).

140. HPS2-THRIVE Collaborative Group. HPS2-THRIVE randomized placebo-controlled trial in 25 673 high-risk patients of ER niacin/laropiprant: trial design, pre-specified muscle and liver outcomes, and reasons for stopping study treatment. Eur Heart J. **34,** 1279-1291 (2013).

141. Roth, E.M., McKenney, J.M., Hanotin, C., Asset, G. & Stein, E.A. Atorvastatin with or without an antibody to PCSK9 in primary hypercholesterolemia. N Engl J Med. **367,** 1891-1900 (2012).

142. Escolà-Gil, J.C. *et al.* Sitosterolemia: diagnosis, investigation, and management. *Curr Atheroscler Rep.* **16,** 424-8 (2014).

143. Patel, S.B. Recent advances in understanding the STSL locus and ABCG5/ABCG8 biology. *Curr Opin Lipidol.* **25,** 169-175 (2014).

144. Hobbs, H.H., Russell, D.W., Brown, M.S. & Goldstein, J.L. The LDL receptor locus in familial hypercholesterolemia: mutational analysis of a membrane protein. *Annu Rev Genet.* **24,** 133-170 (1990).

145. Cuchel, M., Bruckert, E., Ginsberg, H.N. *et al.* Homozygous familial hypercholesterolaemia: new insights and guidance for clinicians to improve detection and clinical management. A position paper from the Consensus Panel on Familial Hypercholesterolaemia of the European Atherosclerosis Society. *Eur Heart J.* **35,** 2146-2157 (2014).

146. Talmud, P.J., Futema, M. & Humphries, S.E. The genetic architecture of the familial hyperlipidaemia syndromes: rare mutations and common variants in multiple genes. *Curr Opin Lipidol.* **25,** 274-281 (2014).

147. Innerarity, T.L. *et al.* Familial defective apolipoprotein B-100: a mutation of apolipoprotein B that causes hypercholesterolemia. *J Lipid Res.* **31,** 1337-1349 (1990).

148. Pullinger, C.R. *et al.* Familial ligand-defective apolipoprotein B. Identification of a new mutation that decreases LDL receptor binding affinity. *J Clin Invest.* **95,** 1225-1234 (1995).

149. Thomas, E.R.A., Atanur, S.S., Norsworthy, P.J. *et al.* Identification and biochemical analysis of a novel APOB mutation that causes autosomal dominant hypercholesterolemia. *Mol Genet Genomic Med.* **1,** 155-161 (2013).

150. Lambert, G., Sjouke, B., Choque, B., Kastelein, J.J.P. & Hovingh, G.K. The PCSK9 decade. *J Lipid Res.* **53,** 2515-2524 (2012).

151. Cohen, J.C., Boerwinkle, E., Mosley, T.H. & Hobbs, H.H. Sequence variations in PCSK9, low LDL, and protection against coronary heart disease. *N Engl J Med.* **354,** 1264-1272 (2006).

152. Talmud, P.J., Shah, S., Whittall, R. *et al.* Use of low-density lipoprotein cholesterol gene score to distinguish patients with polygenic and monogenic familial hypercholesterolaemia: a case-control study. *Lancet.* **381,** 1293-1301 (2013).

153. Filigheddu, Quagliarini, F., Campagna, F. F. *et al.* Prevalence and clinical features of heterozygous carriers of autosomal recessive hypercholesterolemia in Sardinia. *Atherosclerosis.* **207,** 162-167 (2009).

154. Fellin, R., Arca, M., Zuliani, G., Calandra, S. & Bertolini, S. The history of Autosomal Recessive Hypercholesterolemia (ARH). From clinical observations to gene identification. *Gene.* **555,** 23-32 (2015).

155. Remérand, G. *et al.* Four successful pregnancies in a patient with mucopolysaccharidosis type I treated by allogeneic bone marrow transplantation. *J Inherit Metab Dis.* **32 Suppl 1,** S111-3 (2009).

156. Rassoul, F., Richter, V., Lohse, P. *et al.* Long-term administration of the HMG-CoA reductase inhibitor lovastatin in two patients with cholesteryl ester storage disease. *Int J Clin Pharmacol Ther.* **39,** 199-204 (2001).

157. Katulanda, G.W. *et al.* Apolipoproteins in diabetes dyslipidaemia in South Asians with young adult-onset diabetes: distribution, associations and patterns. *Ann. Clin. Biochem.* **47,** 29-34 (2010).

158. Stettler, C., Suter, Y., Allemann, S. *et al.* Apolipoprotein B as a long-term predictor of mortality in type 1 diabetes mellitus: a 15-year follow up. *J Intern Med.* **260,** 272-280 (2006).

159. Bruno, G. *et al.* Effect of age on the association of non-high-density-lipoprotein cholesterol and apolipoprotein B with cardiovascular mortality in a Mediterranean population with type 2 diabetes: the Casale Monferrato study. *Diabetologia.* **49,** 937-944 (2006).

160. Riediger, N.D., Bruce, S.G. & Young, T.K. Cardiovascular risk according to plasma apolipo-protein and lipid profiles in a Canadian First Nation. *Chronic Dis Can.* **31**, 33-38 (2010).

161. Wang, W., Khan, S., Blackett, P., Alaupovic, P. & Lee, E. Apolipoproteins A-I, B, and C-III in young adult Cherokee with metabolic syndrome with or without type 2 diabetes. *J Clin Lipidol.* **7**, 38-42 (2013).

162. Tolonen, N. *et al.* Lipid abnormalities predict progression of renal disease in patients with type 1 diabetes. *Diabetologia.* **52**, 2522-2530 (2009).

163. Hwang, Y.C., Ahn, H.Y., Kim, W.J., Park, C.Y. & Park, S.W. Increased apoB/A-I ratio indepen-dently associated with Type 2 diabetes mellitus: cross-sectional study in a Korean population. *Diabet Med.* **29**, 1165-1170 (2012).

164. Tannock, L.R. & King, V.L. Proteoglycan mediated lipoprotein retention: a mechanism of diabetic atherosclerosis. *Rev Endocr Metab Disord.* **9**, 289-300 (2008).

165. Seo, M.H. *et al.* Association of lipid and lipoprotein profiles with future development of type 2 diabetes in nondiabetic Korean subjects: a 4-year retrospective, longitudinal study. *J Clin Endo-crinol Metab.* **96**, E2050-4 (2011).

166. Hwang, Y.C., Ahn, H.Y., Yu, S.-H., Park, S.W. & Park, C.Y. Atherogenic dyslipidaemic profiles associated with the development of Type 2 diabetes: a 3.1-year longitudinal study. *Diabet Med.* **31**, 24-30 (2014).

167. Ganda, O.P., Jumes, C.G., Abrahamson, M.J. & Molla, M. Quantification of concordance and discordance between apolipoprotein-B and the currently recommended non-HDL-cholesterol goals for cardiovascular risk assessment in patients with diabetes and hypertriglyceridemia. *Diabetes Res. Clin Pract.* **97**, 51-56 (2012).

168. Wild, R.A. Dyslipidemia in PCOS. *Steroids.* **77**, 295-299 (2012).

169. Yin, Q. *et al.* Apolipoprotein B/apolipoprotein AI ratio is a good predictive marker of metabolic syndrome and pre-metabolic syndrome in Chinese adolescent women with polycystic ovary syndrome. *J Obstet Gynaecol Res.* **39**, 203-209 (2013).

170. Roe, A. *et al.* Decreased cholesterol efflux capacity and atherogenic lipid profile in young women with PCOS. *J Clin Endocrinol Metab.* **99**, E841-7 (2014).

171. Kong, X. *et al.* Lipid-lowering agents for nephrotic syndrome. *Cochrane Database Syst Rev.* **12**, CD005425 (2013).

172. Baigent, C. *et al.* The effects of lowering LDL cholesterol with simvastatin plus ezetimibe in patients with chronic kidney disease (Study of Heart and Renal Protection): a randomised placebo-controlled trial. *Lancet.* **377**, 2181-2192 (2011).

173. Prichard, S., Cianflone, K. & Sniderman, A. The role of the liver in the pathogenesis of hyperlipid-emia in patients with end-stage renal disease treated with continuous ambulatory peritoneal dialysis. *Perit Dial Int.* **16 Suppl 1**, S207-10 (1996).

174. Sniderman, A. *et al.* Hyperapobetalipoproteinemia: the major dyslipoproteinemia in patients with chronic renal failure treated with chronic ambulatory peritoneal dialysis. *Atherosclerosis.* **65**, 257-264 (1987).

175. Sniderman, A.D., Sloand, J.A., Li, P.K.T., Story, K. & Bargman, J.M. Influence of low-glucose peritoneal dialysis on serum lipids and apolipoproteins in the IMPENDIA/EDEN trials. *J Clin Lipidol.* **8**, 441-447 (2014).

176. Palmer, S.C. *et al.* HMG CoA reductase inhibitors (statins) for people with chronic kidney disease not requiring dialysis. *Cochrane Database Syst Rev.* **5**, CD007784 (2014).

177. Alam, A., Palumbo, A., Mucsi, I., Barré, P.E. & Sniderman, A.D. Elevated troponin I levels but not low grade chronic inflammation is associated with cardiac-specific mortality in stable hemo-dialysis patients. *BMC Nephrol.* **14**, 247 (2013).

178. Tacikowski, T., Milewski, B., Dzieniszewski, J., Nowicka, G. & Walewska-Zielecka, B. Comparative analysis of plasma lipoprotein components assessed by ultracentrifugation in primary biliary cirrhosis and chronic hepatitis. *Med Sci Monit.* **6,** 325-329 (2000).

179. Ghio, A., Bertolotto, A., Resi, V., Volpe, L. & Di Cianni, G. Triglyceride metabolism in pregnancy. *Adv Clin Chem.* **55,** 133-153 (2011).

180. Retnakaran, R. *et al.* The postpartum cardiovascular risk factor profile of women with isolated hyperglycemia at 1-hour on the oral glucose tolerance test in pregnancy. *Nutr Metab Cardiovasc Dis.* **21,** 706-712 (2011).

181. Bassuk, S.S. & Manson, J.E. Oral contraceptives and menopausal hormone therapy: relative and attributable risks of cardiovascular disease, cancer, and other health outcomes. *Ann Epidemiol.* 2015 Mar;25(3):193-200.

182. Barton, M. Cholesterol and atherosclerosis: modulation by oestrogen. *Curr Opin Lipidol.* **24,** 214-220 (2013).

183. Bassuk, S.S. & Manson, J.E. Menopausal hormone therapy and cardiovascular disease risk: utility of biomarkers and clinical factors for risk stratification. *Clin. Chem.* **60,** 68-77 (2014).

184. Forman, E.J., Guyton, J.R., Filip, S.J. & Price, T.M. Implanted estrogen pellets associated with hypertriglyceridemia, biliary dyskinesia and focal nodular hyperplasia of the liver: a case report. *J Reprod Med.* **55,** 87-90 (2010).

185. Kolovou, G.D., Anagnostopoulou, K.K., Kostakou, P.M., Bilianou, H. & Mikhailidis, D.P. Primary and secondary hypertriglyceridaemia. *Curr Drug Targets.* **10,** 336-343 (2009).

186. Lee, J. & Goldberg, I. J. Hypertriglyceridemia-induced pancreatitis created by oral estrogen and in vitro fertilization ovulation induction. *J Clin Lipidol.* **2,** 63-66 (2008).

187. Henneman, P., Schaap, F.G., Rensen, P.C.N., van Dijk, K.W. & Smelt, A. H. M. Estrogen induced hypertriglyceridemia in an apolipoprotein AV deficient patient. *J Intern Med.* **263,** 107-108 (2008).

188. Goldenberg, N.M., Wang, P. & Glueck, C.J. An observational study of severe hypertriglyceridemia, hypertriglyceridemic acute pancreatitis, and failure of triglyceride-lowering therapy when estrogens are given to women with and without familial hypertriglyceridemia. *Clin Chim Acta.* **332,** 11-19 (2003).

189. Giannarelli, C., Klein, R.S. & Badimon, J.J. Cardiovascular implications of HIV-induced dyslipidemia. *Atherosclerosis.* **219,** 384-389 (2011).

190. Balasubramanyam, A., Sekhar, R.V., Jahoor, F., Jones, P.H. & Pownall, H.J. Pathophysiology of dyslipidemia and increased cardiovascular risk in HIV lipodystrophy: a model of 'systemic steatosis'. *Curr Opin Lipidol.* **15,** 59-67 (2004).

191. Bucher, H.C. *et al.* Small dense lipoproteins, apolipoprotein B, and risk of coronary events in HIV-infected patients on antiretroviral therapy: the Swiss HIV Cohort Study. *J Acquir Immune Defic Syndr.* **60,** 135-142 (2012).

192. de Carvalho, E.H. *et al.* Prevalence of hyperapolipoprotein B and associations with other cardiovascular risk factors among human immunodeficiency virus-infected patients in Pernambuco, Brazil. *Metab Syndr Relat Disord.* **8,** 403-410 (2010).

193. National Cholesterol Education Program (NCEP) Expert Panel on Detection, Evaluation, and Treatment of High Blood Cholesterol in Adults (Adult Treatment Panel III). Third Report of the National Cholesterol Education Program (NCEP) Expert Panel on Detection, Evaluation, and Treatment of High Blood Cholesterol in Adults (Adult Treatment Panel III) final report. *Circulation.* **106,** 3143-3421 (2002).

194. Reiner, Z., Catapano, A.L., De Backer, G. & Graham, I. ESC/EAS Guidelines for the management of dyslipidemia: the task force for the management of dyslipidaemias of the European Society of Cardiology (ESC) and the European Atherosclerosis Society (EAS). *Eur Heart J.* 2011 Jul;32(14):1769-818.

195. Anderson, T.J., Grégoire, J., Hegele, R.A. *et al.* 2012 update of the Canadian Cardiovascular Society guidelines for the diagnosis and treatment of dyslipidemia for the prevention of cardiovascular disease in the adult. *Can J Cardiol.* **29,** 151-167 (2013).

196. JBS3 Board. Joint British Societies' consensus recommendations for the prevention of cardiovascular disease (JBS3). *Heart.* **100 Suppl 2,** ii1-ii67 (2014).

197. Jacobson, T.A. *et al.* National Lipid Association recommendations for patient-centered management of dyslipidemia: part 1 – executive summary. *J Clin Lipidol.* **8,** 473-488 (2014).

197a. Hegele RA, Ginsberg HN, Chapman J, on behalf of the European Atherosclerosis Society Consensus Panel. The polygenic nature of hypertriglyceridaemia: implications for definition, diagnosis, and management. *Lancet Diabetes Endocrinol.* 2014 Aug;2(8):655-66.

198. Sniderman, A.D., Lamarche, B., Contois, J.H. & De Graaf, J. Discordance analysis and the Gordian Knot of LDL and non-HDL cholesterol versus apoB. *Curr Opin Lipidol.* **25,** 461-467 (2014).

199. Contois, J.H. *et al.* Apolipoprotein B and cardiovascular disease risk: position statement from the AACC Lipoproteins and Vascular Diseases Division Working Group on Best Practices. *Clin Chem.* **55,** 407-419 (2009).

200. Takeuchi, T. *et al.* Comparison of cardiovascular disease risk associated with 3 lipid measures in Japanese adults. *J Clin Lipidol.* **8,** 501-509 (2014).

201. Triglyceride Coronary Disease Genetics Consortium and Emerging Risk Factors Collaboration *et al.* Triglyceride-mediated pathways and coronary disease: collaborative analysis of 101 studies. *Lancet.* **375,** 1634-1639 (2010).

202. Jørgensen, A.B., Frikke-Schmidt, R., Nordestgaard, B.G. & Tybjaerg-Hansen, A. Loss-of-function mutations in APOC3 and risk of ischemic vascular disease. *N Engl J Med.* **371,** 32-41 (2014).

203. Varbo, A., Benn, M., Tybjaerg-Hansen, A. & Nordestgaard, B. G. Elevated remnant cholesterol causes both low-grade inflammation and ischemic heart disease, whereas elevated low-density lipoprotein cholesterol causes ischemic heart disease without inflammation. *Circulation.* **128,** 1298-1309 (2013).

204. Sniderman, A.D., Tremblay, A.J., De Graaf, J. & Couture, P. Calculation of LDL apoB. *Atherosclerosis.* **234,** 373-376 (2014).

205. Sniderman, A.D., Williams, K., Contois, J.H. *et al.* A meta-analysis of low-density lipoprotein cholesterol, non-high-density lipoprotein cholesterol, and apolipoprotein B as markers of cardiovascular risk. *Circ Cardiovasc Qual Outcomes.* **4,** 337-345 (2011).

206. Emerging Risk Factors Collaboration *et al.* Major lipids, apolipoproteins, and risk of vascular disease. *JAMA.* **302,** 1993-2000 (2009).

207. Emerging Risk Factors Collaboration *et al.* Lipid-related markers and cardiovascular disease prediction. *JAMA.* **307,** 2499-2506 (2012).

208. Sniderman, A., McQueen, M., Contois, J., Williams, K. & Furberg, C.D. Why is non-high-density lipoprotein cholesterol a better marker of the risk of vascular disease than low-density lipoprotein cholesterol? *J Clin Lipidol.* **4,** 152-155 (2010).

209. Sniderman, A.D., Tremblay, A., De Graaf, J. & Couture, P. Phenotypes of hypertriglyceridemia caused by excess very-low-density lipoprotein. *J Clin Lipidol.* **6,** 427-433 (2012).

210. AACC Lipoproteins and Vascular Diseases Division Working Group on Best Practices *et al.* Association of apolipoprotein B and nuclear magnetic resonance spectroscopy-derived LDL particle number with outcomes in 25 clinical studies: assessment by the AACC Lipoprotein and Vascular Diseases Division Working Group on Best Practices. *Clin Chem.* **59,** 752-770 (2013).

210a. Sniderman, A.D., de Graaf, J., Couture, P. ApoB and the apoB atherogenic Dyslipoproteinemias. In: *The Johns Hopkins Textbook of Dyslipidemia.* Ed: Peter O. Kwiterovich, Wolter Kluwer, China 2009 pp 196-210

211. Lamarche, B. *et al.* Apolipoprotein A-I and B levels and the risk of ischemic heart disease during a five-year follow-up of men in the Québec cardiovascular study. *Circulation.* **94,** 273-278 (1996).

212. Lamarche, B. *et al.* Small, dense low-density lipoprotein particles as a predictor of the risk of ischemic heart disease in men. Prospective results from the Québec Cardiovascular Study. *Circulation.* **95,** 69-75 (1997).

213. Walldius, G., Tchernof A., Moorjani S. *et al.* High apolipoprotein B, low apolipoprotein A-I, and improvement in the prediction of fatal myocardial infarction (AMORIS study): a prospective study. *Lancet.* **358,** 2026-2033 (2001).

214. Sharrett, A.R. *et al.* Coronary heart disease prediction from lipoprotein cholesterol levels, triglycerides, lipoprotein(a), apolipoproteins A-I and B, and HDL density subfractions: The Atherosclerosis Risk in Communities (ARIC) Study. *Circulation.* **104,** 1108-1113 (2001).

215. Expert Panel on Detection, Evaluation, and Treatment of High Blood Cholesterol in Adults. Executive Summary of The Third Report of The National Cholesterol Education Program (NCEP) Expert Panel on Detection, Evaluation, And Treatment of High Blood Cholesterol In Adults (Adult Treatment Panel III). *JAMA.* **285,** 2486-2497 (2001).

216. Sniderman, A.D. *et al.* Concordance/discordance between plasma apolipoprotein B levels and the cholesterol indexes of atherosclerotic risk. *Am J Cardiol.* **91,** 1173-1177 (2003).

217. Cromwell, W.C. *et al.* LDL Particle Number and Risk of Future Cardiovascular Disease in the Framingham Offspring Study – Implications for LDL Management. *J Clin Lipidol.* **1,** 583-592 (2007).

218. Otvos, J.D., Mora, S., Shalaurova, I., *et al.* Clinical implications of discordance between low-density lipoprotein cholesterol and particle number. *J Clin Lipidol.* **5,** 105-113 (2011).

219. Mora, S., Buring, J.E. & Ridker, P.M. Discordance of low-density lipoprotein (LDL) cholesterol with alternative LDL-related measures and future coronary events. *Circulation.* **129,** 553-561 (2014).

220. Sniderman, A.D., Islam, S., Yusuf, S. & McQueen, M.J. Discordance analysis of apolipoprotein B and non-high density lipoprotein cholesterol as markers of cardiovascular risk in the INTER-HEART study. *Atherosclerosis.* **225,** 444-449 (2012).

221. Sniderman, A.D., Islam, S., Yusuf, S. & McQueen, M.J. Is the superiority of apoB over non-HDL-C as a marker of cardiovascular risk in the INTERHEART study due to confounding by related variables? *J Clin Lipidol.* **7,** 626-631 (2013).

221a. Pencina, M.J, D'Agostino, R.B., Zdrojewski, T., Williams, K., Thanassoulis, G., Furberg, C.D., Peterson, E.D., Vasan, R.S., Sniderman, A.D. Apolipoprotein B improves risk assessment of future coronary heart disease in the Framingham Heart Study beyond LDL-C and non-HDL-C. *Eur J Prev Cardiol.* 2015 Jan 29. pii: 2047487315569411. [Epub ahead of print]

222. European Association for Cardiovascular Prevention & Rehabilitation *et al.* ESC/EAS Guidelines for the management of dyslipidaemias: the Task Force for the management of dyslipidaemias of the European Society of Cardiology (ESC) and the European Atherosclerosis Society (EAS). *Eur Heart J.* **32,** 1769-1818 (2011).

223. Stone, N.J., Tchernof, A., Moorjani, S. *et al.* 2013 ACC/AHA guideline on the treatment of blood cholesterol to reduce atherosclerotic cardiovascular risk in adults: a report of the American College of Cardiology/ American Heart Association Task Force on Practice Guidelines. *Circulation.* **129,** S1-45 (2014).

224. Hayward, R. A. & Krumholz, H. M. Three reasons to abandon low-density lipoprotein targets: an open letter to the Adult Treatment Panel IV of the National Institutes of Health. *Circ Cardiovasc Qual Outcomes.* **5,** 2-5 (2012).

225. LaRosa, J.C., Grundy, S.M., Waters, D.D. *et al.* Intensive lipid lowering with atorvastatin in patients with stable coronary disease. *N Engl J Med.* **352,** 1425-1435 (2005).

226. Athyros, V.G. *et al.* Relationship between LDL-C and non-HDL-C levels and clinical outcome in the GREek Atorvastatin and Coronary-heart-disease Evaluation (GREACE) Study. *Curr Med Res Opin.* **20**, 1385-1392 (2004).

227. Downs, J.R. *et al.* Primary prevention of acute coronary events with lovastatin in men and women with average cholesterol levels: results of AFCAPS/TexCAPS. Air Force/Texas Coronary Atherosclerosis Prevention Study. *JAMA.* **279**, 1615-1622 (1998).

228. Nakamura, H. *et al.* Primary prevention of cardiovascular disease with pravastatin in Japan (MEGA Study): a prospective randomised controlled trial. *Lancet.* **368**, 1155-1163 (2006).

229. Post Coronary Artery Bypass Graft Trial Investigators. The effect of aggressive lowering of low-density lipoprotein cholesterol levels and low-dose anticoagulation on obstructive changes in saphenous-vein coronary-artery bypass grafts. *N Engl J Med.* **336**, 153-162 (1997).

230. Cholesterol Treatment Trialists' (CTT) Collaboration *et al.* Efficacy and safety of more intensive lowering of LDL cholesterol: a meta-analysis of data from 170,000 participants in 26 randomised trials. *Lancet.* **376**, 1670-1681 (2010).

231. Toth, P.P., Thanassoulis, G., Williams, K., Furberg, C.D. & Sniderman, A. The Risk-Benefit Paradigm vs the Causal Exposure Paradigm: LDL as a primary cause of vascular disease. *J Clin Lipid.* **8**, 594-605 (2014).

232. Law, M.R., Wald, N.J. & Rudnicka, A.R. Quantifying effect of statins on low density lipoprotein cholesterol, ischaemic heart disease, and stroke: systematic review and meta-analysis. *BMJ.* **326**, 1423-0 (2003).

233. Awan, Z., Seidah, N.G., MacFadye, J.G. *et al.* Rosuvastatin, proprotein convertase subtilisin/ kexin type 9 concentrations, and LDL cholesterol response: the JUPITER trial. *Clin Chem.* **58**, 183-189 (2012).

234. Blazing, M.A., Giugliano, R.P., Cannon, C.P. *et al.* Evaluating cardiovascular event reduction with ezetimibe as an adjunct to simvastatin in 18,144 patients after acute coronary syndromes: final baseline characteristics of the IMPROVE-IT study population. *Am Heart J.* **168**, 205-12.e1 (2014).

235. Sniderman, A., Thanassoulis, G., Couture, P. *et al.* Is lower and lower better and better? A re-evaluation of the evidence from the Cholesterol Treatment Trialists' Collaboration meta-analysis for low-density lipoprotein lowering. *J Clin Lipid.* **6**, 303-309 (2012).

236. Mancini, G.B. J. *et al.* Diagnosis, prevention, and management of statin adverse effects and intolerance: proceedings of a Canadian Working Group Consensus Conference. *Can J Cardiol.* **27**, 635-662 (2011).

237. Rasmussen, J.N., Chong, A. & Alter, D. A. Relationship between adherence to evidence-based pharmacotherapy and long-term mortality after acute myocardial infarction. *JAMA.* **297**, 177-186 (2007).

238. Simpson, R.J. *et al.* Treatment pattern changes in high-risk patients newly initiated on statin monotherapy in a managed care setting. *J Clin Lipid.* **7**, 399-407 (2013).

239. Desai, C.S., Martin, S.S. & Blumenthal, R.S. Non-cardiovascular effects associated with statins. *BMJ.* **349**, g3743-g3743 (2014).

240. Shin, S., Jang, S., Lee, T.-J. & Kim, H. Association between non-adherence to statin and hospitalization for cardiovascular disease and all-cause mortality in a national cohort. *Int J Clin Pharmacol Ther.* **52**, 948-956 (2014).

241. Grundy, S.M., Cleeman, J.I., Merz, C.N. *et al.* Implications of recent clinical trials for the National Cholesterol Education Program Adult Treatment Panel III guidelines. *Circulation.* 2004 Jul 13;110(2):227-39.

242. Boekholdt, S.M. *et al.* Association of LDL cholesterol, non-HDL cholesterol, and apolipoprotein B levels with risk of cardiovascular events among patients treated with statins: a meta-analysis. *JAMA.* **307**, 1302-1309 (2012).

243. Collins, R. *et al.* MRC/BHF Heart Protection Study of cholesterol-lowering with simvastatin in 5963 people with diabetes: a randomised placebo-controlled trial. *Lancet.* **361,** 2005-2016 (2003).

244. Thanassoulis, G., Williams, K., Ye, K. *et al.* Relations of change in plasma levels of LDL-C, non-HDL-C and apoB with risk reduction from statin therapy: a meta-analysis of randomized trials. *J Am Heart Assoc.* 2014 Apr 14;3(2):e000759.

245. Sniderman, A.D. Differential response of cholesterol and particle measures of atherogenic lipoproteins to LDL-lowering therapy: implications for clinical practice. *J Clin Lipid.* **2,** 36-42 (2008).

246. Sniderman, A.D., De Graaf, J. & Couture, P. Low-density lipoprotein-lowering strategies: target versus maximalist versus population percentile. *Curr Opin Cardiol.* **27,** 405-411 (2012).

247. Quirós-Alcalá, L., Mehta, S. & Eskenazi, B. Pyrethroid pesticide exposure and parental report of learning disability and attention deficit/hyperactivity disorder in U.S. children: NHANES 1999-2002. *Environ Health Perspect.* **122,** 1336-1342 (2014).

248. Sniderman, A.D. & Furberg, C.D. Age as a modifiable risk factor for cardiovascular disease. *Lancet.* **371,** 1547-1549 (2008).

249. Sniderman, A.D., Toth, P.P., Thanassoulis, G., Pencina, M.J. & Furberg, C.D. Taking a longer term view of cardiovascular risk: the causal exposure paradigm. *BMJ.* **348,** g3047-g3047 (2014).

250. Goff, D.C. *et al.* 2013 ACC/AHA guideline on the assessment of cardiovascular risk: a report of the American College of Cardiology/American Heart Association Task Force on Practice Guidelines. *Circulation.* **129,** S49-73 (2014).

251. Expert Dyslipidemia Panel of the International Atherosclerosis Society Panel members. An International Atherosclerosis Society Position Paper: global recommendations for the management of dyslipidemia – full report. *J Clin Lipid.* **8,** 29-60 (2014).

252. Heart Protection Study Collaborative Group. MRC/BHF Heart Protection Study of cholesterol lowering with simvastatin in 20,536 high-risk individuals: a randomised placebo-controlled trial. *Lancet.* **360,** 7-22 (2002).

253. Detrano, R.C., Doherty, T.M., Davies, M.J. & Stary, H.C. Predicting coronary events with coronary calcium: pathophysiologic and clinical problems. *Curr Probl Cardiol.* **25,** 374-402 (2000).

254. Pencina, M.J. *et al.* Application of new cholesterol guidelines to a population-based sample. *N Engl J Med.* **370,** 1422-1431 (2014).

255. Davies, M.J. The pathophysiology of acute coronary syndromes. *Heart.* **83,** 361-366 (2000).

256. Kramer, M.C. A. *et al.* Relationship of thrombus healing to underlying plaque morphology in sudden coronary death. *J Am Coll Cardiol.* **55,** 122-132 (2010).

257. Fuster, V., Badimon, L., Badimon, J.J. & Chesebro, J.H. The pathogenesis of coronary artery disease and the acute coronary syndromes (1). *N Engl J Med.* **326,** 242-250 (1992).

258. Kolodgie, F.D. *et al.* Intraplaque hemorrhage and progression of coronary atheroma. *N Engl J Med.* **349,** 2316-2325 (2003).

259. Pencina, M.J., D'Agostino, R.B., Larson, M.G., Massaro, J.M. & Vasan, R.S. Predicting the 30-year risk of cardiovascular disease: the Framingham heart study. *Circulation.* **119,** 3078-3084 (2009).

260. Navar-Boggan, A.M. *et al.* Hyperlipidemia in early adulthood increases long-term risk of coronary heart disease. *Circulation.* **131,** 451-458 (2015).

Printed in the United States
By Bookmasters